W9-ASE-397

Casebook on

the

Termination of

Life-Sustaining Treatment

and

the Care of the Dying

Medical Ethics Series

David H. Smith and Robert M. Veatch, editors

Casebook on the Termination of Life-Sustaining Treatment and the Care of the Dying

EDITED BY CYNTHIA B. COHEN

Indiana University Press • BLOOMINGTON AND INDIANAPOLIS

The Hastings Center • BRIARCLIFF MANOR

Theodore Lownik Library
Illinois Benedictine College
Lisle, Illinois 60532

174.24
C 337

© 1988 by The Hastings Center

All rights reserved

No part of this book may be reproduced or utilized in any form or by
any means, electronic or mechanical, including photocopying and
recording, or by any information storage and retrieval system, without
permission in writing from the publisher. The Association of American
University Presses' Resolution on Permissions constitutes the only
exception to this prohibition.

MANUFACTURED IN THE UNITED STATES OF AMERICA

Library of Congress Cataloging-in-Publication Data

Casebook on the termination of life-sustaining
 treatment and the care of the dying.

 (Medical ethics series)
 Companion v. to: Guidelines on the termination of
life-sustaining treatment and the care of the dying.
 Bibliography: p.
 Includes index.
 1. Terminal care—Moral and ethical aspects—Case
studies. 2. Life support systems (Critical care)—
Moral and ethical aspects—Case studies. I. Cohen,
Cynthia B. II. Guidelines on the termination of
life-sustaining treatment and the care of the dying.
III. Series. [DNLM: 1. Ethics, Medical—case studies.
2. Life Support Care—case studies. 3. Terminal Care—
case studies. W 50 C3373]
 R726.C36   1988   174'.24   88-45101
 ISBN 0-253-31321-X
 ISBN 0-253-21207-3 (pbk.)
 1 2 3 4 5 92 91 90 89 88

Contents

PART ONE:
Making Treatment Decisions
—The Decisionmaking Process

PART TWO:
Specific Treatment Modalities

A. *Long-Term Life-Supporting Technology— Ventilators and Dialysis*

B. *Emergency Interventions—Cardiopulmonary Resuscitation and Life-Threatening Bleeding*

PART THREE:
Prospective Planning: Advance Directives

PART FOUR:
Declaring Death

PART FIVE:
Policy Considerations

A. Ethics Committees

B. Institutional Policies for Patient Admissions and Transfers

C. The Use of Economic Considerations in Decisions
   Concerning Life-Sustaining Treatments

PREFACE

The difficult moral, legal, and social problems created by our increasingly so-phisticated ability to keep people alive have been of special concern to The Hastings Center. As an institute devoted to questions of ethics, particularly those posed by advances in medicine and biology, the center has grappled with the issues surrounding the application of life-sustaining medical technology. To develop responses to these issues the center convened a research group in 1985 whose members were drawn from the fields of medicine, nursing, philosophy, law, and health care administration. As a result of the efforts of this group, the center published a comprehensive set of recommendations, *Guidelines on the Termination of Life-Sustaining Treatment and the Care of the Dying* (Briarcliff Manor, NY: The Hastings Center), in 1987. These are designed to assist health care professionals, patients, and surrogates responsible for making decisions about the use of life-sustaining treatment, as well as policymakers, scholars, and others interested in these issues.

This casebook was developed as a companion to the *Guidelines* to show how clinical cases could be resolved and how the *Guidelines* could be put to work in practice. It presents cases based on actual situations, each of which is followed by a commentary by a member of The Hastings Center research group. The cases focus on such questions as who should make treatment decisions and on what basis; how and when diverse treatment modalities, including respirators, blood transfusions, antibiotics, and pain-relieving drugs, should and should not be used; and whether economic considerations should play a role in decisions to end treatment. The order in which the cases and commentaries appear follows the sequence in which the *Guidelines* address the issues. The book can be used as a separate document that stands on its own or in conjunction with the *Guidelines*. It is meant to be used in educational settings, particularly in medical schools, nursing schools, house officer training programs, continuing education courses for health care professionals, and by ethics committees. This, however, does not preclude its use by others who wish to gain new insights into the issues. Although the cases are based on actual situations, names and facts have been changed in them to preserve confidentiality. Any correspondence to the name of an actual individual in an actual situation, therefore, is purely coincidental. The views expressed in the commentaries are those of the commentators, not of the project as a whole. Indeed, in some instances, commentators may argue a different view.

Warm thanks go to the members of the research group who cheerfully contributed cases and commentaries. Their names are listed in the Contributors section. Susanna E. Bedell, of the East Texas Diagnostic Clinic, also contributed two cases that she encountered in her practice. Special thanks are due to Daniel Callahan, director of The Hastings Center; Susan M. Wolf, Associate for Law at The Hastings Center; and Peter J. Cohen, professor of anesthesiology at the University of Pennsylvania, for editorial and substantive advice that—as usual—was invaluable. Dr. Cohen's poetic endeavors bore fruit in the sonnet in Case 17. The creative writing skills of Elizabeth Carey Cohen, graduate student at the University of Pennsylvania, are responsible for some of the more intriguing parts of the cases. Lou Shenk, fellow in anesthesiology at the University of Pennsylvania, kindly revised Case 18 from a house officer's perspective. Helpful suggestions for the introduction were provided by Linwood Urban, professor of religion at Swarthmore College, and Willard Green, chairman of the Department of Humanities and Social Sciences at Hahnemann University. Janet Bower's nimble mind and fingers put the book into readable shape during times that would have tried the soul of anyone else. Finally, the book would not have been developed without the generous support of Mrs. Shirley Katzenbach, whose continuing interest in the project was a great source of encouragement.

Cynthia B. Cohen

CONTRIBUTORS

Dan W. Brock, Ph.D.
Professor of Philosophy and Program in
 Medicine
Brown University
Providence, RI

Daniel Callahan
Director
The Hastings Center
Briarcliff Manor, NY

Michael C. Cantor, M.D.
Fellow, Division of Digestive Diseases
New York Hospital/Cornell Medical
 Center
New York, NY

Eric J. Cassell, M.D.
Clinical Professor of Public Health
Cornell University Medical College
New York, NY

Cynthia B. Cohen, Ph.D., J.D.
Philosophy Department
Villanova University
Villanova, PA and
Adjunct Associate
The Hastings Center
Briarcliff Manor, NY

Ronald E. Cranford, M.D.
Associate Physician in Neurology
Hennepin County Medical Center
Minneapolis, MN

Harold Edgar, L.L.B.
Julius Silver Professor of Law, Science,
 and Technology
Columbia University School of Law
New York, NY

Lois Evans, D.N.Sc., R.N.
Assistant Professor
University of Pennsylvania School of
 Nursing
Philadelphia, PA

Paul Homer, M.A.
Assistant to the Director
The Hastings Center
Briarcliff Manor, NY

Bruce Jennings, M.A.
Associate for Policy Studies
The Hastings Center
Briarcliff Manor, NY

Joanne Lynn, M.D.
Associate Professor
George Washington University Medical
 Center
Washington, DC

Mathy Mezey, Ed.D., R.N.
Professor of Gerontological Nursing and
Director, The Robert Wood Johnson
 Foundation Teaching Nursing Home
 Program
University of Pennsylvania School of
 Nursing
Philadelphia, PA

David H. Miller, M.D.
Director, Coronary Care Unit and
Assistant Professor of Medicine
New York Hospital/Cornell Medical
 Center
New York, NY

Harry R. Moody, Ph.D.
Deputy Director
Brookdale Center on Aging of Hunter
 College
New York, NY

Ellen Olson, M.D.
Medical Director
Village Nursing Home
New York, NY

Ruth Oratz, M.D.
Division of Oncology
Bellevue Hospital
New York University Medical Center
New York, NY

Robert M. Veatch, Ph.D.
Professor of Medical Ethics
Kennedy Institute of Ethics
Georgetown University
Washington, DC

Susan M. Wolf, J.D.
Associate for Law
The Hastings Center
Briarcliff Manor, NY

INTRODUCTION

Cynthia B. Cohen

The remarkable new means that medical science has developed to prolong human life nurture our hope for immortality. In an earlier era, we accepted death's inevitability and resigned ourselves to comforting those in its grasp. More recently, however, we have refused to accede to our mortality so readily and have attempted to defeat death with the new medical technologies at our disposal. This has been of tremendous benefit to many who are alive today only because of these medical advances. Yet we are learning that our burgeoning medical powers over death can also prolong a painful process of dying for some and return others to what they consider a living death of a kind unknown to previous generations. Mindful of Prometheus, who brought fire to humans from the gods only to be chastised for his pride, we search for the wisdom to know when and how to temper our technologically-driven passion for immortality.

Some question the benefit of automatically providing patients near death with life-sustaining treatment. They believe that we should accept the biblical concept of a "time to die" and refrain from keeping people alive in conditions that destroy human dignity and augment suffering. Others ask whether we can financially afford an ethos that encourages us to do everything possible to save patients from death. Economic factors, they maintain, push us toward ending aggressive treatment of patients whose care is expensive and whose chances for recovery are small. Still others argue that we must do everything possible to keep patients alive or else risk a devaluation of human life that is contrary to our most basic communal values. The shadow of the Nazis casts its pall.

A virtual explosion of debate has taken place in recent years about how we should meet such conflicting individual and societal values when we confront decisions to withdraw or to withhold life-sustaining treatment. There is a pressing need to establish a coherent policy that will assist us to make these difficult choices in ways that reflect the core values and preferences of patients, the conscientious beliefs of health caregivers, and the great moral weight that our society places on human worth, individual autonomy, and social justice. In response to this need, a Hastings Center research group developed *Guidelines on the Termination of Life-Sustaining Treatment and the Care of the Dying* (Briarcliff Manor, NY: The Hastings Center, 1987), which drew on the vast literature that has developed on this topic and on the specialized knowledge of research group members. The *Guidelines* provide a basic format for decisionmaking in these difficult situations and then range over the use of such treatment modalities as respirators, blood transfusions, antibiotics, and pain-relieving drugs. They also address basic policy issues such as whether economic considerations should enter decisions to end treatment and the role that institutional ethics committees should play in such decisions.

Ethical values are at the heart of the *Guidelines*. Yet ethical guidelines are not moral blueprints. For this reason, the *Guidelines* suggest basic ways in which to respond to the issues at stake consistent with the ethical framework at the foundation of our society that must then be adapted to the specific problems at hand. This requires skill at recognizing when an ethical issue has arisen, determining which ethical values and principles apply, how conflicts between these can be resolved, what choices between available options are ethically viable, and what the comparative consequences of the implementation of these choices would be.

Many health care professionals do not feel prepared by their education to deal with these challenges. Physicians, nurses, and allied health professionals have been trained to view medicine and nursing as forms of science. And science, they have been taught, is value-free. Yet they find that the practice of medicine and nursing is not only scientific, but fraught with values. They have been taught that the relationship between the health care professional and the patient is inviolable. Yet they must frequently face the reality that hospital administrators, third-party payors, and malpractice litigators impinge on this relationship. They have been taught that economic considerations should not enter into treatment decisions. Yet they are pressured to recognize such considerations on a daily basis. Health care professionals who must reconcile requirements to be objective scientists, compassionate caregivers, and economic gatekeepers face major quandaries. As a consequence, physicians, nurses, and other health caregivers have increasingly come to recognize the importance of proficiency at ethical, as well as medical, diagnosis. Although particular ethical problems that they encounter in the clinical situation are often subject to clear resolution on a "rule of thumb" basis, at times more difficult issues arise that require them to consider ethical values and principles themselves. Health care professionals realize that reliance on quick and easy solutions to complex ethical problems is likely to be unsatisfactory and that those who have thought about such questions before a crisis are more likely to find an adequate solution to them.

A major purpose of this book is to facilitate the efforts of health care professionals and students to hone their clinical ethical skills as they deal with the perplexing issues related to stopping or withholding treatment. It should also be useful to patients, families, surrogates, public officials, and others who deal with these ethical issues. The case study approach is familiar to students and teachers in the various professions. It is grounded in the view that theoretical knowledge can be better understood and integrated through application to specific patient care situations. This approach also provides a ready way for those who are not acquainted with the concrete realities of the health care system to learn about how these affect the resolution of difficult ethical questions that arise in practice. For these reasons, this method was adopted in this book.

Although the cases presented here are based on actual situations, they have been modified to protect the confidentiality of those involved. Some are oriented toward particular treatment modalities and to the clinical context in which decisions about their use are made, since the setting in which care is provided itself affects the range of medical and moral alternatives available. Others are directed toward policy governing the amount and kind of health services available, for this, too, influences decisions about forgoing life-sustaining treatment and the care of the dying. The commentaries refer to specific sections of the *Guidelines*. These references are set within brackets. This casebook need not be used in conjunction with the *Guidelines,* although it is hoped that the cases will stimulate readers to consult them.

Any meaningful ethical inquiry must examine and challenge deeply held beliefs and customary values. The purpose of ethical reflection is not only to find solutions to moral problems in health care that respect individual beliefs, the traditions of the health care professions, and the shared values of the moral community, but to question these when they are in conflict or appear misdirected. Readers may see things differently from the commentators or from their fellow readers. Should this occur, it would confirm, rather than undermine, the usefulness of this casebook, for the book is meant to help readers develop the faculty of ethical reflection, rather than eliminate the need for it.

No cases and commentaries can displace careful deliberation by those involved in making difficult ethical choices about the use of life-sustaining treatment. They can, however, assist health care professionals, patients, and others to develop an ethical framework that will serve them in good stead, not only in the specific circumstances under consideration in the cases, but in other contexts as well. Our novel power to keep patients alive, like the newly discovered fire of Prometheus, offers us opportunities to extend and enrich human life that were not even conceived of in previous eras. It offers, as well, opportunities to gain new insight into our basic values and to reaffirm our commitments to respect human life, individual autonomy and dignity, and social justice.

Part One

Making Treatment Decisions —The Decisionmaking Process

1. Whose Decision?
The Case of Roy Gantos

Roy Gantos lay in his hospital bed and indicated repeatedly to his nurses, doctors, and relatives that he no longer wanted to be maintained on a ventilator. He did this in written statements ("Don't prolong my life") and by frantically shaking his head, "No," to questions about whether he wanted to remain on the machine. Four months earlier he had been admitted to the hospital for back pain and leg weakness. At that time, the fifty-eight-year-old man was diagnosed as having squamous cell carcinoma of the hypopharynx (cancer of the throat) for which little could be done. He had been sent home, but metastases were noted in his lungs and liver at a check-up, revealing that the cancer had spread, and he had been readmitted to the hospital.

Surgery on Mr. Gantos one day after his second admission confirmed that he had widespread cancer of the spinal cord with localized compression at the midthoracic level. The pressure on his spinal cord was relieved by the surgery, but he had to be placed on a ventilator due to a combination of problems, including severe chronic obstructive lung disease and recurrent episodes of pneumonia. Attempts to wean him from the ventilator were unsuccessful. After four weeks, Mr. Gantos began to indicate clearly to doctors and nurses that he did not want to remain on the ventilator.

Mr. Gantos's closest relatives, a brother and a nephew who lived with him, felt that he should be removed from the ventilator. They told Dr. Swisher, Mr. Gantos's physician, that they had viewed a television program together in which a legal deposition was taken from a California man who wanted to be removed from a ventilator. He, like Mr. Gantos, had chronic obstructive pulmonary disease. In addition, he suffered from inoperable cancer of the lung, an abdominal aneurysm, and heart problems. He, too, could not be weaned from the ventilator. When they saw him on T.V., he was lying in an Intensive Care Unit bed with his hands tied down by his sides and was supported by various technological devices. They watched him shake his head, "No", to the question whether he wanted to continue on the ventilator. Yet when he died, he was still being maintained on the machine. The final court decision, which held that he had the right to refuse such treatment, had come too late for him. Mr. Gantos had told his brother and nephew that if he ever became so ill that there was little hope for his recovery, he would not want to be maintained by a machine like that.

Dr. Swisher, however, believed that if the ventilator were kept in place and he provided vigorous treatment, he could keep his patient alive for several months. He explained this to Mr. Gantos's brother, and told him that he doubted that Mr. Gantos had the capacity to make a decision at this time. He thought that he was suffering from "ICU psychosis", a severe disorientation brought on in some patients by the intensive care setting and regimen. Only the week before, Dr. Swisher recounted, he had cared for a patient who had become very depressed on readmission to the ICU who asked that he not receive life-prolonging treatment. Dr. Swisher overruled this request when the patient suffered a heart attack, and ran a "Code" on him that saved his life. When the patient recovered, he thanked Dr. Swisher profusely, and this had convinced the doctor that critically ill patients could not make good decisions for themselves. He believed that he should do everything possible to save them, regardless of their statements to the contrary.

Who should make the decision about whether to remove Mr. Gantos from the ventilator? What procedures would you recommend for determining the appropriate decisionmaker? What standard for making the decision should be used?

Commentary by Susan M. Wolf

The central question in this case is who should decide whether to remove this critically ill patient from the ventilator: the physician, the patient, or the patient's family. Resolving that question will determine whether the ventilator is withdrawn. Dr. Swisher believes that he should make the decision and would refuse to remove the patient from the ventilator. Mr. Gantos himself has previously expressed his preference not to be maintained on a ventilator in this state and now reaffirms this in the ICU. Mr. Gantos's closest relatives believe that the patient's wish should be honored and that he should be removed.

Dr. Swisher's prior experience, in which he overruled a patient's refusal of life-prolonging treatment and the patient later thanked him, has persuaded him to overrule all critically ill patients' refusals of such treatment. But the doctor is overinterpreting a single case; he assumes that because one patient gave thanks, all would. We know this is not the case. An empirical study of resuscitation has demonstrated that many patients who are not given an opportunity to refuse resuscitation regret having been resuscitated. Moreover, the single case Dr. Swisher focuses on is one in which the patient recovered. In many cases the use of life-sustaining treatment will not lead to recovery. Instead, the patient will find the treatment a burden that prolongs pain and suffering. In Mr. Gantos's case, recovery is not even a possibility—Dr. Swisher expects the ventilator at best to prolong the patient's life for several months.

Most importantly, Dr. Swisher's inclination to make the treatment decision himself denies the patient any role in the decisionmaking process. In the name of doing what he thinks best for the patient, he would take away the patient's moral and legal right to determine for himself what is best and to refuse invasive treatments. In the name of paternalism he would rob the patient of autonomy.

Decisions about the use of life-sustaining treatment cannot be the physician's sole prerogative. The physician and patient each have a critical role to play in the decisionmaking process. The physician brings his or her medical expertise, past experience, and compassion to bear; the patient brings his or her own sense of values and priorities. Neither alone has an adequate basis for a decision. The physician's information, support, and advice allow the patient to apply the patient's own values to determine whether several more months of life on a ventilator offer benefits and opportunities for satisfaction that outweigh the burdens. These are personal and individual decisions—one patient may leap at any opportunity for more time, while another may not want a few more months of life on a ventilator. By determining to ignore those patients who wish to forgo life-sustaining treatment, Dr. Swisher forces one choice on them all.

In this case, Dr. Swisher has doubts that Mr. Gantos has the capacity to make the decision in the ICU, because Mr. Gantos seems to be suffering from "ICU psychosis." In order to make decisions about their care, patients must have decisionmaking capacity—the ability to understand information given to them, reflect on it in accordance with their values, and communicate their decision. The fact that a patient is under stress and reacting to confinement in the ICU does not necessarily mean that he has lost those functional abilities. Dr. Swisher needs to assess carefully whether the patient has lost decisionmaking capacity and, if so, whether anything can be done to restore that capacity to an adequate level.

In the event that the physician remains persuaded that the patient lacks capacity and that no corrective action is possible, the next question is who should assume the effective decisionmaking role. Someone must act as a substitute decisionmaker for the patient—ideally someone who knows the patient's values and preferences and can bring them to bear in collaborating with the physician. In this case the patient's closest relatives are well suited to be his surrogates. Not only have they lived with him, but Mr. Gantos has actually discussed with them his preferences about ventilator use. Because the nephew and brother are in agreement, it is unnecessary to choose between them and identify a single surrogate.

The final major question is what standard the surrogates should apply in deciding about the ventilator. When surrogates make decisions about a patient's care, their goal should be to decide as the patient would if he were able. They are acting as the patient's agents, asserting for him his right to refuse treatment. In this case, it is clear what the patient would want; he stated his preference earlier, before his decisionmaking capacity became questionable. He is reaffirming that preference now. The physician's doubts about the patient's current decisionmaking capacity raise questions about how much weight should be accorded to his current statements. Because his prior preferences are known, however, it is not necessary to clarify how much weight should be given to his current statements; the important fact is that he is affirming, rather than contradicting, his prior preferences.

Dr. Swisher should regard Mr. Gantos's brother and nephew as surrogate decisionmakers. However, because Mr. Gantos can still participate in the decisionmaking process, he should be involved in the process too, even though he may not be capable of exercising full decisionmaking authority. All should consult together. Because the surrogates believe the ventilator should be removed in accordance with the patient's prior preference and the patient concurs, the ventilator should be removed. Dr. Swisher should examine his resistance to this and might find it helpful to clarify his reservations with colleagues or the institution's ethics committee, if there is one. If in the last analysis, Dr. Swisher feels that as a matter of conscience he cannot comply with the patient's and surrogates' decision, then he should so notify them. If they then wish to transfer to another physician, Dr. Swisher should assist in that process.

This analysis is in accord with the recommendations of the *Guidelines*. The "Guidelines on the Decisionmaking Process" in Part One depict a partnership between doctor and patient—the physician does not arrogate decisions about the use of life-sustaining treatment to him- or herself, and the patient does not make decisions in lonely isolation. Instead, they collaborate, the physician applying his or her expertise and the patient bringing to bear his or her values, to make the ultimate determination of whether to accept the treatment offered.

When the patient lacks decisionmaking capacity, the *Guidelines* recommend that one or more surrogate decisionmakers—usually those closest to the patient—exercise the ultimate decisionmaking authority, trying to decide as the patient would. If the patient has left clear instructions, written or verbal, those should be honored. [*See* Part One, II., (3) "Identifying the key decisionmaker," (b) "Identifying a surrogate," and (4) "Making the decision," (c) "The patient who lacks decisionmaking capacity."]

If the physician has strong reservations about acting in accordance with the patient's or surrogate's decision, consultation with the ethics committee, as recommended in the *Guidelines*, may prove useful. The *Guidelines* recognize, however, that in some cases a physician will feel unable to comply with the patient's or surrogate's decision. In those cases the *Guidelines* recommend that the physician notify the decisionmaker of the problem and partici- pate in an orderly transfer of the patient to another physician, if that is the pa- tient's or surrogate's wish. [*See* Part One, II., (8) "Objections and challenges," (e) "Withdrawal of health care professional or institution."]

2. A Question of Capacity:
The Case of Megan O'Rourke

Megan O'Rourke, a seventy-year-old widow, lived in a nursing home. Although she was sometimes confused and disoriented about the time and where she was, she was aware of much of what was happening to her and was responsive to it. Generally she complied with simple suggestions and fed and dressed herself. Bathing and grooming were a little more difficult, and she required some assistance with these. Her caregivers viewed her as a generally pleasant and cooperative person who would, on occasion, express her dislike of a situation by grimacing and turning away with several firm shakes of her head. Once or twice a month, her daughter, who lived nearby, came to visit her.

Mrs. O'Rourke had severe emphysema that required careful medication and oxygen therapy. She also had arteriosclerotic heart disease and symptomatic congestive heart failure. A stroke had left her with both receptive and expressive aphasia (an inability both to understand language and to express herself verbally) and with minor right-sided motor weakness (incomplete paralysis of her right side).

Three months ago, during an episode of acute bronchitis, a chest X-ray was taken of Mrs. O'Rourke, and a solitary pulmonary nodule indicated that she might have lung cancer. Nursing home caregivers discussed a further work-up, including bronchoscopy (a procedure in which an observation tube is inserted into the windpipe under local anesthetic), with her daughter, as they did not believe that Mrs. O'Rourke had the capacity to make her own decisions. Her daughter, however, refused bronchoscopy on grounds that it was an invasive and somewhat risky procedure that would cause her mother discomfort. Her mother was treated with oral antibiotics and oxygen by nasal cannula for her bronchitis and returned to baseline within a week.

Last week, Mrs. O'Rourke was extremely short of breath, feverish, and in more severe congestive heart failure. She was brought by ambulance to the Emergency Room of the nearby hospital. Medical evaluation revealed that she was in pulmonary edema, hypoxic, and probably infected. She was admitted to the Intensive Care Unit of the hospital after stabilization in the Emergency Room. The leading diagnosis was lung cancer with pneumonia and exacerbation of both chronic obstructive pulmonary disease and congestive heart failure.

Members of the house staff told Mrs. O'Rourke's daughter that they wanted to perform bronchoscopy through the endotracheal tube in order to make a more definitive diagnosis. They explained that her treatment would be different if she had small cell rather than squamous cell lung cancer. Small cell lung cancer is significantly more responsive to chemotherapy than squamous cell lung cancer—partial or complete remissions are not uncommon. They felt that Mrs. O'Rourke's clinical status and sense of well-being could be improved if she had small cell lung cancer and responded to chemotherapy.

Mrs O'Rourke's daughter refused bronchoscopy for her mother and rejected the possibility of chemotherapy. However, she insisted that "everything else be done" for her, including prolonged intubation and placement in the Intensive Care Unit with full resuscitative efforts and use of vasopressors if necessary.

Mrs. O'Rourke's own preference was unclear, as was her capacity to make a decision. Members of the house staff considered taking one of the following courses of action:

a) following the wishes of Mrs. O'Rourke's daughter;

b) consulting Mrs. O'Rourke herself, and giving her the benefit of the doubt about the question of capacity;

c) going to the hospital ethics committee;

d) contacting the hospital legal counsel;

e) treating her as they thought best.

Should they follow one of these or some other course? What factors weigh most heavily for and against your recommendation?

Commentary by Dan W. Brock

The central issues of this case are whether the patient has the capacity to participate with her physician in making decisions about her treatment, and, if she does not, who should decide for her and by what standards. She is described as having been sometimes confused and disoriented to time and place when in the nursing home and as suffering from receptive and expressive aphasia resulting from a stroke. Her caregivers in the nursing home do not believe that she has the capacity to make her own decisions. On the other hand, she is described as generally aware of much of what is happening to her, responsive to it, and able to comply with simple suggestions and to express her dislike of a situation. Mrs. O'Rourke thus falls into that large class of patients of questionable competence.

The first responsibility of the health care team is to assess the patient's capacity to make the decisions now at hand—whether a diagnostic bronchoscopy will be done and whether, if it is determined that the patient has a small cell lung cancer, she will undergo chemotherapy. Some commentators hold that decisionmaking capacity is a *global status* true of all patients in certain general categories. Increasingly, however, decisionmaking capacity is understood to be *decision specific,* meaning that in cases of uncertain or borderline capacity the patient may be able to make some decisions but not others because of their differing demands. The patient's capacity to make the specific decisions at hand must be assessed.

This initially may involve using simple tests of Mrs. O'Rourke's understanding and memory, such as are part of crude screening devices like the Mini Mental Status Exam. Unless such tests unequivocally establish her near-complete inability to understand and reason in even the simplest situations, however, the health care team should attempt to explain in terms likely to be understandable to Mrs. O'Rourke the nature of her medical condition and of the decisions that must be made. Decisionmaking capacity requires that Mrs. O'Rourke have not merely the ability to understand this information, but also the ability to deliberate about the choice in terms of her own preferences and values and to communicate her choice to others. Mrs. O'Rourke's aphasia will inevitably make the assessment of her capacity difficult. All possible means of facilitating her ability to understand, choose, and communicate her wishes need to be utilized. For example, it may well be necessary to communicate with her in writing and for her to respond in writing. It is quite likely that, even if Mrs. O'Rourke is able to communicate her wishes, there will still be significant uncertainty about how much and how well she understands. This will raise the question of what level of decisionmaking capacity should be required for Mrs. O'Rourke to be accepted as having the capacity to make the decision.

Some commentators have argued for a *fixed* standard of capacity, usually understood as a threshold level of understanding that the patient must have to be deemed to have capacity. Among those who argue for a fixed standard there is disagreement about how high the standard should be set. At one extreme is the requirement that the patient merely be able to express a preference for one alternative. At the other extreme are standards that apply some "objective" criterion of the "best" alternative, which is independent of the patient's own settled aims and values.

Other commentators have argued in favor of a *variable* standard of capacity. The more the patient's choice appears to be contrary to his or her best interests, the higher the level of understanding and reasoning that the patient should display, and the greater the certainty of the evaluator that that level is attained by the patient. The rationale behind the variable standard is that it should balance respecting people's right to decide for themselves when they are able to do so against protecting them from the harmful consequences of their choices when their decisionmaking capacities are seriously impaired. Thus, the more contrary to their well-being patients' choices appear to be, the higher the level of decisionmaking capacity, as well as certainty that that level is attained, it is reasonable to require.

Since Mrs. O'Rourke's serious cardiac and pulmonary disease indicate that she has limited life expectancy and her condition is extremely discomforting and seriously compromises the quality of her remaining life, whether a bronchoscopy is done and chemotherapy provided will not make a substantial difference to her well-being. Hers are circumstances in which many persons, indeed perhaps most, would choose not to undergo chemotherapy for any form of lung cancer unless it would clearly enhance their comfort. Therefore, most would choose not to undergo diagnostic procedures useful only if treatment is being considered. Consequently, whether her choice is to consent to bronchoscopy and chemotherapy or to refuse them, this is not a case in which to insist on more than a moderate standard of capacity. She should probably be given the benefit of at least some doubt if she is able to express her wishes about treatment at all.

Another controversial aspect of the capacity question is whether final determination about her capacity to decide can be made by her responsible physician, in this case apparently the house staff, or whether it is necessary to appeal to the courts for a formal determination of her competence.

If the house staff judge her to have the capacity to make her own choice and her daughter disagrees, attempts should be made to resolve the disagreement. Whatever informal means are available and appropriate should be utilized, such as bringing in psychiatric consultants on the patient's capacity, social workers, clergy, and others. If necessary, more formal means may be employed such as referral to an ethics committee or ultimately to the courts. A patient with decisionmaking capacity, however, retains authority to decide about his or her health care, and no consent from family members is required.

If, on the other hand, the house staff concur with the nursing home personnel and the daughter that Mrs. O'Rourke is incompetent to decide, most commentators would agree that there is a strong presumption that a family member who knew her best should be her decisionmaking surrogate. (In some cases, though not apparently in this one, the potential surrogate who knew the patient best may not be a family member.) Few, if any, would hold that house staff may simply treat her as they think best.

An issue of some controversy, however, is by what standards the daughter should decide and whether she should have the same range of discretion the patient would. Most commentators hold that the daughter should employ the so-called *substituted judgment* standard, which requires the surrogate to attempt to decide as the patient would have decided if she had capacity. The point of this standard is to allow the surrogate to make use of any knowledge of the patient's wishes and values relevant to the decision at hand.

Those who reject the substituted judgment standard usually favor instead the so-called *best interests* standard, which uses some more "objective" criterion of what treatment is "best" in the circumstances. It is one responsibility of the house staff to help ensure that the daughter is making her decisions on the basis of an appropriate standard.

The particular choices of the daughter—refusing consent to bronchoscopy or chemotherapy, while insisting on other aggressive measures to sustain life, including prolonged ventilator support, ICU care, and CPR—raise the issue of the extent to which patients or their surrogates should be permitted to "pick and choose" some treatments while rejecting others. Hospital policies now increasingly make clear that a Do Not Resuscitate order should be compatible with a full range of other treatment measures. Thus, patients or their surrogates should have the discretion to decide about the particular treatments necessary to best tailor the overall treatment plan to the patient's values and wishes.

The daughter's decisions in this case, however, raise a question about whether a coherent treatment approach is being pursued. For example, the bronchoscopy was first rejected because it would be invasive, risky, and discomforting to the patient. With the patient now intubated, so that the bronchoscopy could be performed through the endotracheal tube, some of these objections are removed. Nevertheless, doing the bronchoscopy to make a more definitive diagnosis of the lung cancer may still be unwarranted if the daughter has categorically rejected chemotherapy to treat the cancer. What needs further exploration is whether diagnosis and chemotherapy treatment of Mrs. O'Rourke's lung cancer, if it is of small cell type, would be compatible with keeping her mother as comfortable as possible. Given Mrs. O'Rourke's multiple and grave illnesses, the house staff also have a responsibility to discuss further with her daughter whether aggressive measures such as prolonged intubation, ICU care, and CPR would have been wanted by, or are in the best interests of, her mother in these circumstances. The house staff should combine considerable flexibility in following the patient's or surrogate's decision with her responsibility to ensure that apparently problematic or inconsistent decisions really do meet the wishes or best interests of the patient.

The *Guidelines* also understand capacity not as a general status of the patient, but as situation specific and requiring, in cases of questionable capacity, an assessment in the decision at hand. [*See* Part Six: "Special Problems," III. "Decisionmaking capacity and competence."] The *Guidelines* reject an outcome standard that looks only to the content of the choice made. Instead, they adopt a process standard that requires the responsible health care professional to assess the patient's exercise of her decisionmaking capacities in the decision in question. The *Guidelines* adopt the variable level standard of capacity that requires a higher level of capacity the more harmful to the patient his or her choice appears to be. They accept the idea that the more that is at stake for the patient in terms of harm produced or benefit lost in her choice, the higher the level of capacity, as well as certainty that the level is attained, that should be insisted on. This variability is necessary to give due weight to protecting the patient from the harmful consequences of her choice.

The *Guidelines* also address the selection of a surrogate and the standards by which a surrogate should decide. [*See* Part One, II., (3) "Identifying the key decisionmaker," (b) "Identifying a surrogate," and (4) "Making the decision," (c) "The patient who lacks decisionmaking capacity."] They endorse, in the absence of a contrary prior designation by the patient, turning to the person who knew the patient best, usually a family member. The *Guidelines* recommend the *substituted judgment* standard for decisions—using what is known of the patient's preferences and values to try to choose as the patient would have wanted. Helping family members to understand the choice in these terms not only best respects the patient's self-determination, but also can help ease the emotional burden of decisionmaking for family members by leaving responsibility for the choice, as much as is possible in the circumstances, with the patient.

Finally, the *Guidelines* make clear that unless there is irresolvable disagreement among the physician, patient, and surrogate about either the patient's capacity or the treatment alternative chosen (including the alternative of no life-sustaining treatment), there is no necessity for further consultation with an ethics committee or adjudication by the courts. Resort to these bodies in general should be reserved for cases where serious conflict or uncertainty persists about how to proceed.

Part Two

Specific Treatment
Modalities

3. Communication Problems:
The Case of Horace Berlin

Horace Berlin, a determined seventy-two-year-old retired business executive, has had severe chronic obstructive pulmonary disease for many years. His most recent hospitalization for respiratory failure (there have been three) was in Florida, four months ago. He hated the whole business—the respirator, the treatments, the bed rest, even the nurses buzzing around him all the time. He hated it so much, in fact, that he finally gave up smoking. When he came back home to New York City, he was supposed to see a physician whose name he had been given by his Florida doctor, but he put it off. Instead, he continued on the medications he had been taking and talked the pharmacist into refilling the prescriptions. He lacked energy. Walking, or any exertion at all, was a problem for him because of shortness of breath—a problem that became slowly but progressively worse after he arrived back in New York.

Three weeks ago Mr. Berlin came down with a cold, and within a few days he was so short of breath that he could hardly walk across the living room. Despite his wife's pleas, he still refused to go to the doctor. The day that he was admitted to the hospital, he awoke with a high fever and finally agreed to get help. After hearing his symptoms over the telephone, the doctor met him in the Emergency Room and promptly admitted him to the Intensive Care Unit. His pCO_2 was 90mm Hg and his pO_2 was 48mm Hg. In addition to his respiratory problems, he was confused and intermittently aware of his confusion. He kept asking his wife, who had not left his side since they entered the Emergency Room, to answer the doctor's questions.

In addition to steroids, antimicrobials, bronchodilators, and fluids, he was put on a respirator. His fever and blood gases quickly responded. He remained intermittently confused, although he knew where he was and why. The attending physician informed his wife that although he seemed to be improving, there was a high probability that he would not be able to be removed from the respirator. She was not surprised, she said, because of what the doctor in Florida had told both of them would happen if "he didn't take care of himself." After a week, an attempt was made to wean him from the respirator, but it did not succeed. Two days later the house staff tried again. Again he deteriorated.

The attending physician kept Mrs. Berlin informed of all the events. At this time, he told her that he believed her husband should be withdrawn from the respirator and that if he could not be maintained without it, he should not be returned to it. The physician made it clear to Mrs. Berlin that her husband would die if he could not breathe on his own without a respirator. Mrs. Berlin responded that she knew that this was coming and that she hoped that all the paraphernalia would be cleared away from the bed so that she could sit with her husband until he died.

The house staff discontinued the respirator, but when Mr. Berlin became dyspneic, they put him back on. When the attending physician learned of this and questioned the house staff, the resident told him that Mrs. Berlin did not really understand what was going to happen. Further, the resident stated, she told him that she wanted her husband continued on the respirator. According to the resident's report, this must have occurred shortly after the attending physician and Mrs. Berlin had agreed to remove her husband from the respirator. The Senior Unit physician, whom the attending physician next questioned, told him that "the lights in the ICU are too bright to be discontinuing respirators and allowing patients to die."

Later that day, Mrs. Berlin asked the attending physician when her husband would be disconnected from "all those machines."

Why did these difficulties about Mr. Berlin's treatment arise? What do you think should have been done instead?

Commentary by Eric J. Cassell

Deciding when a respirator should be discontinued is a frequent problem that may be extremely troubling. The reasons lie in the technology itself, its impact on patients, and the setting in which it is deployed. An inability to maintain blood levels of oxygen sufficient to support consciousness occurs commonly in advanced chronic lung disease and in congestive heart failure and less often in a number of other potentially reversible states. In these conditions, adequate blood oxygen levels can be quickly and easily achieved by current respirators. The technology is universally available in modern hospitals and can be operated safely and without great difficulty. When respirators are appropriately employed, lung function can be supported until the underlying disease is better, at which time patients can be removed from respirators, leaving them unharmed. Although some patients find them unendurable, most tolerate them well. This discussion is concerned with respirators for which intubation or tracheostomy is required and *which do not permit otherwise independent existence.*

Patients whose underlying disease is no longer reversible and who will *not* return to self-sufficiency can be maintained on respirators for prolonged periods—sometimes many months. This category is exemplified by patients with late state chronic pulmonary diseases such as emphysema. For such patients the respirator is necessary to maintain life, but it does not promise or permit a return to any degree of independent living. In other instances, such as far advanced heart failure, the respirator is only one part of more complex life support mechanisms, but it is often the most visible and symbolic expression of their condition. The status of these patients is ambiguous. They are alive, but they cannot expect ever again to do the things that they associate with being alive. They are totally and absolutely dependent on their caregivers for everything. They are bed-bound, and even the actions of their bodies and their field of vision are limited. They cannot eat. If they are intubated, the tube in their mouth (or nose) and throat is a source of variable distress. Things cannot get better.

In the United States, virtually all such patients are treated in Intensive Care Units. In many teaching hospitals their care is under the direction of the physicians in charge of the unit whose expertise is in intensive care (critical care) medicine. Here, the patients' attending physicians operate in an advisory capacity only and are not permitted to write orders or exercise the authority their patients believe is vested in them. In teaching hospitals, the immediate care is usually rendered by house staff, with an intern or first-year resident directly responsible for the patient. The result of this staffing pattern is that in an emergency, when the decision to start or not start a patient on a respirator must be made immediately, it is frequently the responsibility of the most junior physician. The same physician will be the one who discontinues the respirator if that judgment has been made.

The patients on respirators exemplified by this care are alive and can frequently communicate to some degree. It is often difficult, however, to assess such patients' capacity for self-determination, particularly since they rarely know what symptoms or suffering to expect if the respirator is discontinued. If they are removed from the respirator they will surely die, although in what period of time—minutes or hours—may be unclear. It inevitably appears to caregivers that if they remove such patients from their respirators, the caregivers have surely killed them. For that reason, assurances that removing life support is morally the same as not starting it are not comforting. Families faced with the decision to discontinue respirators are in the same position of believing that it is their decision that will cause the patients' deaths—that they have killed them. [*See* Part Six: "Special Problems," I. "Terminating treatment, active voluntary euthanasia, and assisting suicide."]

The problems associated with discontinuation of respirator support arise, then, from their ubiquity and ease of use, their effectiveness in supporting lung function, their lack of harm in appropriate cases, the ambiguous status of patients who cannot live without them, staffing patterns of intensive care units (particularly the fact that the burdens associated with starting or stopping respirators most often fall on the most inexperienced physician), difficulties in determining the patient's capacity to make decisions, and finally, the illusion—difficult to deny—that it is not the underlying disease that kills the patient but the person who discontinues the respirator.

Because of all these considerations, the vital question is not whether the respirator will support lung function, since that is almost always the case. Rather, *the most important determination to be made before starting a respirator is the degree of probability that the patient can ever be successfully removed from it.* In trauma or postoperatively, or in diseases such as pneumonia, pulmonary emboli, acute heart failure, acute lung failure, or acute decompensation of chronic lung disease secondary to infection, the probabilities are that the patient will be independent of the respirator when the acute condition has cleared. The possibility, if true, that the underlying condition will worsen and that the patient may never be able to live free of the respirator must be mentioned in discussions with the patient and family or when obtaining consent. Further, plans should be made at the time of consent for such an eventuality.

Where the probability is high that the patient will never again be able to function free of the respirator, the physician obtaining consent should not emphasize the rare possibility of ultimate independent survival, but stress the problems to be faced in the *likely* event that the patient will *not* survive weaning from the respirator. In such cases it should be made clear at the outset that if the patient cannot live independently of the respirator, he or she will nevertheless be removed from it. At that time it should be stressed that the patient will not be allowed to suffer in coming off the respirator. If it becomes necessary to remove the patient under these conditions, maintaining high flow of oxygen by mask (it is hypoxia that causes distress), allowing CO_2 to build up, and utilizing adequate sedation with morphine and/or diazepam will keep the patient comfortable until death. Appropriately managed, death under these conditions can be comfortable and easy for the patient, while affording the family the opportunity of being present at a defined, expected, and peaceful end, unencumbered by the usual paraphernalia and bustle of Intensive Care Units.

In the case at hand, the previous history of the illness gave both the physician and the patient and his wife reason to suspect that he would never be able to come off the respirator. It is unlikely, because of Mr. Berlin's hypercapnia, that the doctor was able to talk about the issues with him. The doctor was apparently frank, however, in discussing the possibility with Mr. Berlin's wife. Despite the good response with the respirator, the physician continued to prepare the wife for the eventuality that Mr. Berlin would not again be able to live off the respirator. It is essential that some long-term view of the problem be maintained with both patients and their families to avoid their becoming either overly optimistic or pessimistic. This does not require the doctor to be omniscient, but merely aware and communicative of the prognostic probabilities. While physicians often become impossibly vague in these circumstances, claiming that they do not wish to be held to their predictions in view of the uncertainties of disease, they must be sympathetic to patients' needs for information. Patients and their families are aware that the doctor's best guess is vastly better than the patient's endless uncertainties.

In view of the fact that the doctor had prepared Mrs. Berlin for her husband's death, why was there such an appearance of vacillation and failed communication between her and the doctors? Often, what appears to be poor communication is, in reality, an unwillingness to accept the consequences of the original conclusion. If, as the attending physician claimed, Mrs. Berlin understood and accepted the need to remove Mr. Berlin from the respirator, then Mr. Berlin would, in fact, have to come off the respirator and die. It is clear from the comments of the Senior Unit physician that the doctors are uncomfortable with this outcome. Further, as the case is presented, it is the resident who will have the task of discontinuing the respirator. We do not know whether he or she has had experience or training in taking people off respirators so that they can die. The metaphor of "pulling the plug" has been used so much that the resident may have that incorrect idea of how it is done. The most probable explanation for the seeming communication problem with Mrs. Berlin is a communication problem among the staff. Cases like this should be handled by full discussion among the members of the ICU, *including the nurses*. The discussion should include the techniques used for discontinuance of respirators, the likely outcomes, and the problems that arise with the patient and the family. *It should never be the responsibility of the most junior or inexperienced member of the medical team to discontinue a respirator in these circumstances. A more experienced or senior physician should always be available.*

The way in which Mr. Berlin was cared for is in general accord with the recommendations of the *Guidelines*—up to the point at which the decision of his surrogate had to be carried out. Although he knew that he might well encounter major medical difficulties and seemed a forceful person who would want to make his own treatment decisions, he made no advance plans in case of an emergency, as recommended by the *Guidelines*. [*See* Part Three: "Prospective Planning, Guidelines on Advance Directives."] His wife, therefore, had to decide for him at a time at which he apparently was unable to make his own choice about whether the ventilator should be withdrawn. It seems safe to conclude from the closeness that they displayed that Mrs. Berlin knew her husband's preferences and values and was trying to choose as he would. [*See* Part One: "Making Treatment Decisions," II. (4) "Making the decision," (b) "The patient whose capacity is fluctuating or uncertain."]

The decision to remove the ventilator was not made unilaterally by the medical staff, but in consultation with Mr. Berlin's surrogate, a practice strongly supported by the *Guidelines*. [*See* Part Two: "Specific Treatment Modalities," Section A, II; "Guidelines on ventilators."] There will always be ways to skirt carrying out a decision that is painful for all, such as those employed in this case, that no guidelines can anticipate and prevent. Greater communication and discussion provide the best way to prevent this.

Problems like the case of Mr. Berlin are not rare and will probably become increasingly common. Hospitals, and particularly Intensive Care Units, should prepare for them by appropriate staff education and technical training. When physicians and nurses have been adequately trained and prepared, cases such as this may be sad or unfortunate, but will not be beyond their technical or personal abilities. It is essential that whether a patient lives or dies, the survivors feel that both technical excellence and compassion marked the care.

4. Ethics or the Law?

The Case of Susan Pagari

Susan Pagari, a fifty-eight-year-old widow, began to notice that she had little appetite and was progressively losing weight. She went for a medical examination in mid-December and had a barium enema that showed a malignant-appearing sigmoid colon lesion. Although a biopsy was negative for colon malignancy, a liver-spleen scan was compatible with cancer, and she was admitted to the hospital for treatment.

X-rays showed that she had an obstruction of her colon. When she was advised to have surgery to remove this, Mrs. Pagari said that she wanted to defer it for several days until the end of the year, so that if she did not survive, her children would not have to pay taxes for the current year on her large estate. She also said that if she had an incurable malignancy, she did not want to receive aggressive treatment or be sent to the Intensive Care Unit.

On December 31, Mrs. Pagari was wheeled into the operating room. During surgery, she was found to have a large malignant tumor of the transverse colon that had spread within the abdominal cavity and had reached her liver. A palliative resection of the transverse colon was performed. The surgery was complicated, and she received massive blood transfusions. Her post-operative course was stormy, and she required ventilatory support.

Mrs. Pagari was placed in the Intensive Care Unit, where she initially improved. On the fifth post-operative day, however, she suffered a heart attack. A Swann-Ganz catheter was passed to monitor her cardiac function and dopamine was instituted to raise her blood pressure, which had dropped precipitously. She was transferred to the Cardiac Care Unit after she went into severe pulmonary edema. Although she responded to fluid restriction and diuresis in the CCU, she pulled out her endotracheal tube and suffered a cardiac arrest. She was resuscitated and improved sufficiently during the next twenty-four hours to allow the dopamine to be discontinued. She was partially weaned from the respirator.

At this time, her daughter and son-in-law met with the physicians and said that they wanted no further life-sustaining treatments for Mrs. Pagari, since her cancer was incurable and she did not appear to have long to live. They believed that she had deliberately extubated herself and that this was in keeping with her no-nonsense, practical nature. They maintained that her desire not to receive intensive care should be respected. The physicians agreed with them, and wrote a "DNR" order. However, they told the family that, as a matter of hospital policy, the respirator could not be discontinued. All tests were minimized, and Mrs. Pagari was kept as comfortable as possible.

The next day, the physicians learned that Mrs. Pagari's son-in-law, who was an attorney, was in the process of seeking a court injunction in order to have the respirator removed. He was also threatening to follow this with a suit against them for arbitrarily overriding Mrs. Pagari's wishes and violating her right to refuse treatment. The physicians contacted the hospital's legal counsel, who advised them that discontinuation of the respirator might prompt the district attorney to seek a murder indictment against them.

Should the respirator be removed? What factors do you think should enter into this decision?

Commentary by Harold Edgar

We come to the case late in the day. We are not told whether Mrs. Pagari is now competent or, if not competent, whether she is sentient. Why was she resuscitated? Why was she sent to the ICU? Did the physicians start down the treatment path with no thought of following her wishes? Was there any doubt about whether her cancer was "incurable," as she had used the term? Did she understand her medical situation better than she did the tax consequences of dying rich in December, about which she was wrong? Was she told the hospital's policy about respirators? Did she agree to it?

Physician-patient relationships are contractual ones. Individuals have no duty to purchase or submit to medical procedures, and their right to choose for themselves comprehends the right to choose what kinds of medical services they want. Physicians have corresponding rights, although less sharply defined ones, to refuse to contract if the patient wants futile or unprofessional services. This contractual view of the matter increasingly represents the dominant American perspective on medical relations. Mrs. Pagari has, on these premises, the right to decide whether and to what extent she wants aggressive medical treatment. It seems as though her wishes have been disregarded at several points.

The fact that respirators are involved does not matter in principle. Ventilation, even if life-saving ventilation, is a form of medical treatment. In these circumstances, does the respirator's use provide what Mrs. Pagari considers a benefit? It seems not, although I would not treat her pulling out the tube as affirmative evidence of that point without much more detail. Nor is there any ethical line worth drawing between terminating a respirator's use and not starting it in the first place. Mrs. Pagari is entitled to have the values by which she lived respected.

Why does the hospital lawyer counsel caution? Five years ago the answer would have been obvious. Respirator technology brings the contract model of medicine directly into conflict with our traditional rules for giving meaning to the sanctity of life, a central value in the Judeo-Christian tradition. In this view, people should die when they must, not when they want to. Life is God's gift and his to reclaim when he chooses. Our criminal law was shaped by this earlier and absolute understanding of the sanctity of life. The traditional rules have never been repealed. You break the criminal law if you intentionally shorten another's life by even a moment. If, for example, somebody jumps from an airplane without a parachute and is sure to die when he hits the ground, and I shoot and kill him before he hits, costing him some thirty seconds of life, I am guilty of criminal homicide in every state in the land. How can these rules admit the permissibility of turning off Mrs. Pagari's air supply?

In earlier times, medicine was shielded from conflict with the criminal law by its perceived impotence, not by a theory of contractual absolution. The patient's disease killed him, not the treatment or lack thereof. Moreover, people died at home. Physicians had no warrant to seek them out. The new medical technology brings people to the hospital to die. And modern medicine makes the timing of death a matter for human choice, not God's. These new realities make conceptual tools like causation and liability for omissions, the law's old favorites, seem wholly unsatisfactory as a basis for distinctions they earlier explained. Who can blame doctors and nurses if they feel personally implicated in the death by asphyxiation of a person who died when he had days of life to go? They see the unresolved conflict between different norms and are not shielded from it, when respiration is involved, by time or physiological uncertainty as to the mechanism by which death occurred. That is why respirators raise special problems.

Nonetheless, there can no longer be any question that our society and our law reject technological vitalism in treating the terminally ill, and that the contract model has triumphed at the points where it overlaps with criminal law norms. We do not violate the sanctity of life when we limit technology's use to settings where it can provide benefit, understood as such, by those we claim to help. A consensus can be found on this point in medical ethics literature of nearly all stripes, in national commissions, in documents like the *Guidelines,* and in the case law of every state whose highest court has considered the matter.

The contract model empowers Mrs. Pagari to decide her treatment. Unfortunately the model does not capture very well the real nature of the actual human interchanges it purports to characterize. It serves best as a tool to limit a tradition of professional control, rather than as a working description of human behavior. For most people in most contract settings do not *want* to exercise their theoretical power to control precisely what they purchase. One of the great myths of liberal thought is that more choice brings more satisfaction. Observe us when we engage lawyers, dry cleaners, or plumbers. We pay people to exercise discretion on our behalf because we do not want to take the trouble to inform ourselves. Indeed, that is precisely what we are paying *them* for, their knowledge of the ways things are ordinarily done. We accomplish this by implicitly granting our agents authority ample to our ends. No one urges us to seize control of these transactions.

It may be argued that health stands in an entirely different relationship to the person than most of the other things we bargain to secure. Even if this is true, the point surely is a double-edged one, for health holds this position precisely because it is linked to our deepest fears about death. I am convinced that most people do not want to engage in a prolonged discussion of the possible meaning of every aberrant test result. One of the things physicians do is take onto themselves the anxiety of worrying about which of the possible explanations for our complaints is the real one and spare us, until it is necessary, the burden of thinking that our troubles are severe. When they are severe, however, it may be excruciatingly difficult to have the necessary conversation or to know what the patient's answers mean.

The contract model, however, assumes the possibility of meaningful physician-patient communications at a morally relevant time, even as it disregards the transaction costs of arranging them—let alone who will pay those costs. Further, its adherents then suppose that, in times of crisis, people on the outside will be confident that a patient's "wishes" are being followed, even though the contract was not witnessed and was made with a person in fear of her life. One can understand the D.A.'s skepticism.

The most satisfactory way to resolve the social problem, I believe, lies in the direction these *Guidelines* point, namely to standardize over time a few basic options and secure their consideration before, not after, serious health problems begin.

The title of this case misleads us because it suggests that medical professionals must frequently choose between performing morally right acts and complying with the law. I do not believe that this proposition is true. Ethics and law, more pointedly medical ethics and law, are not competing world views. Nor do they trigger different considerations that must somehow be balanced one against the other in deciding how to proceed in particular cases. In fact, the law goes almost 180 degrees the other way. It seeks out and ordinarily gives practical effect to medical professionals' opinions about the right way to handle human dilemmas that arise in medicine. This approach is built into the structure of many legal rules, particularly and obviously those such as the malpractice rules, which measure physician performance by whether it matched what similarly-situated physicians do. More importantly for readers of this volume, the courts' opinions show that judges read the bioethics literature and regard it as legally relevant. They accept professional medical consensus at nearly every turn. Physicians are understandably frustrated by legal regulation of medical practice. When it comes to medical ethics issues, however, they vastly underestimate their professional power to shape the rules that apply.

The conflict between individual physicians' moral intuitions and practical lawyers' advice is a much more serious problem. In the Pagari case, the facts are sketchy. Let us suppose, nonetheless, that the physicians have no doubt that Mrs. Pagari wants immediate cessation of ventilation. Lawyers say this may provoke a murder indictment. How should we think about this sort of conflict?

Making predictions is the bedrock art of both medical and legal practice. Yet practicing lawyers, no less than physicians grappling with medical uncertainty, must frequently give advice when they do not know what the law is or how it will be applied to a particular set of facts. Courts solve new cases by finding analogies to old ones; yet there are many competing sources of analogy. Moreover, facts are chancy. How confident can you be that a future judge or a jury—a group of citizens chosen because of their ignorance of the human activities you plan to describe to them—will see the facts as you see them?

Practicing professionals, whether physicians or lawyers, respond similarly to situations where they must advise despite their ignorance. First, they give advice that tries to minimize the likelihood of worst case outcomes, even though following the advice is painful or inconvenient. Patients are told to submit to more tests; clients to prepare more elaborate documents. Second, professionals hide from their clients how ignorant they really are. There are echoes of this in the Pagari case. "The hospital's legal counsel . . . advised them that discontinuation of the respirator might prompt . . . a murder indictment." Are we in a state that has had *no* law or lawsuits on death and dying? Has anyone talked to the district attorney? Or does this advice, like so much legal advice, originate from a simple decision procedure: if one path is almost surely safe and the other potentially risky, take the surely safe path. That way, the adviser need not confront or reveal his own inability to calculate closely what the real risks are and can never be shown to be wrong. Here the chances of a successful tort suit by the son-in-law are low, with little precedent for a substantial damage award. If another child appears and doubts the mother's wishes were correctly understood, might that not lead to a much more expensive suit? Who knows, but why risk it?

There is a rich literature on physicians' responses to uncertainty; less has been written about lawyers'. Their responses, however, are not completely parallel. In medicine, the person most severely affected by the physician's management of uncertainty is the patient herself. She can theoretically demand that *her* preferences be respected. In contrast, lawyer's advice to the client ordinarily involves the way the client treats other people. Because the lawyer's obligation is to protect the client, his or her tendency is to ignore the interests of the others, except to the extent the client's rational self-interest demands otherwise.

When physicians seek legal advice about managing relations with patients, the harm done by this tendency of lawyers is intensified, because physicians cannot treat patients as "others" whose interests are to be accounted for solely in terms of minimizing legal risk. Physicians are bound to patients by precisely the principles of medical ethics the courts are inclined to respect. Thus, when push comes to shove, the question is whether physicians are professionally obligated to run increased legal risks if practicing good medicine requires it. Are they morally obliged to bet on the proposition that ultimately law will respect, and shape itself to embody, any sound principle of medical ethics? I believe they are. The question becomes, however, how much must they bet and how confident should they be that they are *right* in their understanding of what sound principles of ethics require before they are obliged to bet? No simple formula can provide an answer.

The *Guidelines* strongly favor following the wishes of patients with capacity to decide about the use of life-sustaining treatment for themselves. Although we would need further evidence about Mrs. Pagari's abilities to comprehend information, deliberate about choices, and communicate before we felt confident that she had the capacity to make her own treatment decisions [*See* Part Six: "Special Problems," III. "Decisionmaking capacity and competence"], at the time that she rejected aggressive treatment should her cancer prove incurable, there was no reason given to set aside the presumption that she had capacity. We know that Mrs. Pagari's malignancy is incurable in the opinion of her surgeon, for her resection is palliative, not therapeutic. Even so, the provision of intensive care for her might be justifiable as one of those exceptional situations mentioned in the *Guidelines* "when intensive care may provide a form of palliation or pain relief" for patients with irreversible illness who are near death and consequently might not conflict with her wishes. [*See* Part Five: "Policy Considerations," Section B. "Guidelines on institutional policies for patient admissions and transfers," II. (5) "Intensive care units," (a) "Admissions."] However, Mrs. Pagari's poor status after the five day postoperative period in the ICU provides strong evidence that she could not be brought around and that she was in an incurable condition. Palliation within an ICU no longer seems justifiable. In such a case, according to the *Guidelines*, arrangements should have been made, with the concurrence of her surrogate, to remove her from intensive care and to provide her with supportive care.

The hospital, however, has adopted a policy of refusing to discontinue respirators, and the matter is soon to go to court. The physicians should not preempt judicial action, I believe. This is in accord with the recommendations of the *Guidelines*, for the situation has progressed to a point at which an institutional resolution of the issues is no longer possible.

5. Pirate's Beer:
The Case of Richard Fallon

Seventy-four-year-old Richard Fallon used to claim that he was a retired pirate who loved to climb high on the mast of his ship and bellow out over the sea. He explained to others in the Dialysis Unit that his kidney problem was "caused by drinking too much of that dark pirate's beer." He had met his wife while on a voyage to Japan, he would relate to them. He had called to her lustily from the mast as his ship neared shore, and she had boldly approached him when he landed. Shortly afterward, they were married in Buddhist ceremony and had been together ever since.

Four years ago, Mr. Fallon was diagnosed as having kidney failure, and he began hemodialysis. He also had arteriosclerotic heart disease, chronic obstructive pulmonary disease, and multiple episodes of chronic bronchitis. He was rejected for transplantation because of his debilitated condition and his generally uncooperative attitude. Home dialysis had been attempted, but it was unsuccessful due to marital discord. Mr. Fallon was very demanding and even belligerent at times, and his wife could not overcome the many difficulties involved in dialyzing him. Consequently, he was treated at a hospital dialysis unit.

Two years ago, Mr. Fallon had a massive stroke that left him with an expressive aphasia (an inability to express himself verbally) and a right hemiplegia (paralysis of the right side). After the stroke, his course was very rocky. Over a period of several weeks, he showed some signs of improvement. Physical therapy was given to him in the hospital, but with minimal success. He was placed in a nursing home where it was hoped that he could regain sufficient neurologic function to return home. However, he had severe adjustment problems in the nursing home and was transferred back to the hospital for care several times when the staff found him very difficult to treat. Three months after the first stroke, he suffered another in the same hemisphere and became comatose. At that time, his wife asked that no further medical interventions be initiated. Shortly after, however, he regained consciousness and returned to approximately the same level of neurologic function that he had had before the second stroke. He was again discharged to the nursing home.

Currently, Mr. Fallon receives maintenance dialysis treatment in the hospital unit. He is very demanding of staff time; one nursing person must be at his bedside throughout the dialysis. This affects the quality of care provided to other patients in the unit. He has been reevaluated neurologically, and it is considered that he is unlikely to improve much beyond the present point. He will require permanent custodial care. His sensorium is reasonably clear, although he has trouble expressing his thoughts and communicating with others. He no longer mentions pirate's beer.

Because of the likelihood that Mr. Fallon will require permanent custodial care, the Patient Selection Committee has been asked to discuss his case. There is a possibility that dialysis therapy will be discontinued for him, and that he will be allowed to die of uremia. Should this be done?

Commentary by Bruce Jennings

The ethical significance of this case does not reside in the ethical dilemmas or conflicts among principles that it poses. Instead, the case is instructive and raises an ethically significant issue because it focuses our attention on two very different kinds of justifications for forgoing life-sustaining treatment, in this case dialysis.

The first type of justification is patient-centered. It holds that it is ethically permissible to forgo life-sustaining treatment when the experience of continued treatment and the experience of prolonged life with incurable disease and progressive debilitation are intolerably or unreasonably burdensome to the patient.

This is the most commonly discussed and most widely accepted form of justification in the professional literature on the ethics of terminal care. It establishes a weighty burden of argument on those who would favor the termination of treatment, especially when the patient lacks decisionmaking capacity, cannot communicate his or her own wishes, values, or quality of life assessment, or when the patient has not prepared any type of advance directive to guide treatment decisions. But when the burden of argument set up by this type of justification is met, then most people would probably feel reasonably satisfied that the decision to allow the patient to die is based on solid ethical grounds.

The second type of justification is not patient-centered, but is oriented toward the interests and welfare of others who are affected by the patient's treatment and continued life. It holds that it is ethically permissible to forgo life-sustaining treatment when that treatment and the custodial care that must accompany it are unduly or disproportionately burdensome to others.

This second type of justification is much more controversial and problematic than the patient-centered type of justification. It is problematic because it may involve the subordination of the patient's individual rights and interests to considerations of social utility or administrative expedience. This line of reasoning also asks physicians and other health care professionals to look beyond the specific needs and interests of an individual patient and to take a broader view of the social consequences of treatment decisions. Many health care professionals and ethicists are leery of this approach. Government or hospital policymakers may choose not to provide certain services or to limit general patient access to certain treatments in accordance with uniform and equitable criteria. All health care systems must be selective and must inevitably allocate scarce resources in these ways. But when a treatment is generally available to other patients with a similar medical need, should providers at the bedside limit an individual patient's access to that treatment solely on the basis of third-party interests or on the basis of economic or institutional efficiency?

The case of Richard Fallon requires that we distinguish these two types of justification for the termination of treatment. Which type of justification is the most pertinent to the facts of this case? And how would each type of justification unfold when applied to the case?

As the case is presented, it directs our attention to the second type of justification for the termination of treatment. Mr. Fallon's quality of life and the burden imposed by dialysis on *him* are not the focal concerns of his wife (the surrogate), the nursing home and hospital staffs, or the dialysis unit's Patient Selection Committee. Instead, their concerns focus on the burdens Mr. Fallon's care imposes on others—and on themselves. Mr. Fallon is a "problem patient"; his behavior is difficult to manage; worse still, an attendant must be at his bedside throughout the dialysis, and this affects the quality of care being provided to other patients on the unit. Can these facts be used to justify withholding further dialysis from Mr. Fallon—presumably against his will, for he has never indicated his desire to end these treatments—and allowing him to die of uremia?

Here it is instructive to contrast dialysis with access to transplantation and with triage criteria used to determine access to an Intensive Care Unit. When a resource is inherently scarce and is not routinely made available to all who could benefit from it, then a given patient's potential to benefit from the resource may be weighed against the potential benefit to other patients who are competing for the same resource. In determining that Mr. Fallon was not a candidate for transplant, for example, physicians made a classical triage judgment of just this sort: Mr. Fallon's debilitated condition and his uncooperative attitude made it unlikely that he would tolerate the transplant and make a good recovery; in other words, his potential to benefit from a transplant was below a reasonable threshold and did not compare favorably with the potential to benefit other candidates waiting in the queue.

Can the same line of reasoning be used to deny Mr. Fallon access to dialysis? In my judgment, the answer is no. In the 1960s when dialysis machines were a scarce resource akin to donor kidneys, dialysis treatment was subject to allocation based on triage principles. The ethical dilemmas of rationing were overwhelming because most candidates for dialysis could not be screened out on the basis of medical criteria alone. Highly subjective and discriminatory judgments based on the "social worth" of individual patients were made. With the advent of the End Stage Renal Disease Program, the federal government made a public policy decision to take dialysis out of the realm of triage rationing of this kind. Of course, some shortages and utilization pressures continue to affect individual dialysis units, some patients must be referred elsewhere or scheduled at inconvenient times, and so on. But under current circumstances it is surely incorrect to say that because Mr. Fallon is given access to dialysis treatment, some other patient must be denied access. And absent that kind of zero-sum dilemma, the balance between Mr. Fallon's interests and the interests of other patients tips in Mr. Fallon's favor. None of the third party interests affected in the case is strong enough to justify denying Mr. Fallon access to dialysis and allowing him to die.

Now let us consider briefly the bearing that a patient-centered justification for the termination of treatment may have on the case. It is, I think, more difficult to rule out a justification for forgoing dialysis along these lines, and it is this that the decisionmakers in the case ought really to be concerned with. Nonetheless, without a clearer indication of Mr. Fallon's own wishes in the matter, I do not think that a surrogate would be warranted in deciding against continued dialysis under the current circumstances of the case.

Richard Fallon has come a long way since the days when he used to call to young women from atop his ship's mast. From what the case tells us of his life, it is clear that he always hated to be tied down. He was zealously independent, a lover of adventure, a teller of tall tales—in short, the kind of man who has become increasingly marginal and obsolete in our bureaucratic, rule-entangled, institutionalized society. Now, in the twilight of his life, the edifice of his former self-identity and way of being in the world has been chipped away, bit by bit. Chronic debilitating diseases and multiple system failures have sapped his vitality. Aphasia has silenced his stories and robbed him of the capacity of narration, a uniquely significant human power which, evidently, was one of Fallon's principal ways of relating to others. And physical paralysis has done something that social mores and conventions heretofore had not been able to do: it has tied him down.

Hobbled thus by various infirmities, the confining grip of institutions—the hospital, the nursing home, the supervision of his wife during home care—has finally caught up with him. Symbolically, for many patients, and seemingly for Fallon too, the experience of dialysis treatment represents this tethering, this confinement. Given his chronic obstructive pulmonary disease it seems likely that he will also be caught in the net of the ventilator somewhere down the road; and given his behavior, physical restraints await him in the nursing home and on the dialysis unit. But despite having his speech, his physical prowess, and his independence stripped away, something of his old irascible self-identity remains. For that residual self the meaning of all the other restrictions he has suffered, all the other assaults on his self-identity and independence, come together in his dialysis.

Although prolonged dialysis can have many debilitating and unpleasant side effects, there is no indication in this case that the dialysis treatment in and of itself is unduly burdensome to Mr. Fallon, or that he perceives it to be so. And his underlying experience of continued life, despite his many ailments and disabilities, is not meaningless (to him) or fraught with unbearable pain and suffering. In short, this case does not indicate the conditions required by the patient-centered justification for the termination of treatment.

The *Guidelines* generally counsel against an appeal to third-party interests in making decisions to forgo treatment, unless those interests are factored in by the patient himself or herself. Patients with decisionmaking capacity may consider the economic costs and the psychological burdens imposed on their family and loved ones when assessing the benefits and burdens of their continued treatment and the prolongation of their lives. But the *Guidelines* permit surrogates much less latitude in this regard. Both surrogates and health care providers are consistently instructed to promote the patient's well-being and to assess the benefits and burdens of life-sustaining treatment from the patient's own perspective. [*See* Part One: "Making Treatment Decisions," II., (1) "Underlying ethical values," and (4) "Making the decision," (c) "The patient who lacks decisionmaking capacity."]

The *Guidelines* recognize that considerations of justice or equity in the allocation of scarce resources may constrain the patient's right to demand certain forms of treatment and that they must be weighed alongside the obligation of providers and surrogates to respect patient self-determination and to promote patient well-being. But the *Guidelines* generally address these considerations at the policy level and reject them in decisionmaking at the bedside. [*See* Part Five: "Policy Consideration," Section C. "The use of economic considerations in decisions concerning life-sustaining treatments."]

6. "But He Never Told Me Not To": The Case of Jim Adams

The acquired immune deficiency syndrome (AIDS) has proven uniformly fatal. For this reason, the staff—attendings, house staff, nurses, and others—of the AIDS Long-Term Care Unit of City General Hospital was extremely uncomfortable about constantly resuscitating patients with AIDS whom they knew were going to die soon. The patients also were aware of their outlook, and a number of them told doctors and nurses that they did not want to be resuscitated. Consequently, as a matter of policy in the AIDS Unit, the staff began to discuss with each patient admitted whether or not that patient wanted to be resuscitated. The patient's decision was entered on his or her chart.

Jim Adams was admitted to the AIDS Unit at City General before this policy was implemented. Unfortunately, when the policy was in effect at a later time and the staff came to discuss the matter with him, he was suffering from AIDS-related dementia that rendered him unable to make a decision about resuscitation.

In addition to the central nervous system disease, Mr. Adams had all the other problems common to the disease—Kaposi's sarcoma, pneumocystis pneumonia, extensive candidiasis, cryptosporiodosis, and severe diarrhea. He had been resuscitated twice and was now comatose and on a respirator. Severe renal failure had supervened, and his physician was planning to start dialysis. When a nurse asked him why Mr. Adams was going to be dialyzed, the physician responded that he had no other choice, since Mr. Adams had not refused to be resuscitated.

Should dialysis be initiated for Mr. Adams because he never said that he did not want to be resuscitated?

Commentary by Eric J. Cassell

The reason for starting dialysis on Jim Adams, it appears, is that he was not able to tell his doctors not to dialyze him. Because of the concentration on the patient's right to refuse treatment that is found in the *Guidelines,* one might conclude erroneously that treatment is the necessary and automatic response to any disease state, unless the sick person states otherwise. Perhaps it appears that the *Guidelines* are saying that nothing should be done for a sick person except in response to that person's stated autonomous wishes. That is not the case and is very different from saying that nothing should be done *against* the patient's stated autonomous choice. The *Guidelines* are attempting to make explicit that what the patient wants is another crucial factor, that must, in addition to the precepts that have always guided medical action, be taken into account in any medical decision. [*See* Introduction, III. "The ethical framework."]

This is important to clarify since "what a patient wants" is a phrase that bothers physicians because it seems to them to have the force of whim. It sounds like desires that might go this way or that in some unpredictable mode that is hardly of sufficient importance to determine the manner in which patients and physicians engage in struggles with disease, fate, or death. Autonomy is not simply the spoken expression of a person's desire. It has the force of the *continuing* expression of the person. Persons expressing their autonomous decisions are choosing their *future,* not merely their present circumstances. Within the constraints of fate, the future that autonomous persons choose is expected to be consonant with their past choices. The way that they dress, speak, choose, value, and act toward others, objects, events, and relationships in the future can be expected to be in accord with those same behaviors in their past. Because it is difficult for physicians (or others) to know all of this about their patients, the stated desires of patients are taken to represent their autonomous decisions. In most situations such spoken choices, especially if they are developed in a dialogue with the caregiver, can be accepted as the voice of the patient's self-determination.

In circumstances where patients cannot speak for themselves, or where sickness or medical care distort the expression of a person, it is *essential* to search out the person's "voice" in other ways or from other sources. In the *Guidelines,* the use of surrogates for the patient has been extensively discussed, but the presumed voice of the patient can also be found in the tradition of medicine. This tradition demonstrates that the physician is also considered to have a choice in any medical action and that the doctor's choices are meant to be in the best interests of the patient (as the patient would have defined them), even when the patient lacks the capacity to speak.

To see how tradition provides guidance in the case of Jim Adams, let us start with the precepts that guide *any and every therapeutic act,* whether it be an emergency, the start of life-sustaining treatment, or even trivial therapy. The first prerequisite for any treatment, apart from simply the person's desire, is that a sickness is present—there must be suffering, distress, a bodily complaint, interference with function, or the person's belief that he or she is ill. The second prerequisite is that the physician concurs that a reason exists for treatment—there is a diagnosable state that explains the patient's reason for asking for treatment. Other stipulations must be met. These are that a treatment exists; that more good than harm is anticipated; that the physician is not asked to do damage, harm normal tissue, or be a probable cause of death (as in high risk surgery); and finally, that the person is able to ask for the treatment (indeed, the patient is expected to volunteer, albeit with varying degrees of enthusiasm). The tradition acknowledges that the patient must have the capacity to decide.

Medical custom also speaks directly to the case of Jim Adams in its response to emergency situations where a patient is unconscious. It is presumed by the community, not the doctor alone, that the sick person would want to have his or her life saved even if the person cannot at that moment express that desire. Even in emergency circumstances, however, the presumption that a doctor should treat a person rests not only on the immediacy of the need for treatment, but also on the fact that other conditions are met. First, the essence of the situation is its immediacy—it is an event, a complete circumstance of its own in which a medically recognizable problem exists which, if not immediately treated, would lead to permanent disability or death. Second, treatment is possible, or at least offers some promise of reversing the cause of the acute situation. Third, the treatment will not do harm. Fourth, the probability (or at least a reasonable possibility) is that the treatment will permit a viable person to emerge at the other end of the acute situation. In trauma, for example, no one would transfuse a person whose skull had been crushed, even though serious blood loss has been documented and transfusion would restore the blood volume.

In the case of Jim Adams, only some of these conditions are met. While a treatment, peritoneal dialysis, exists, the treatment offers *no* chance of reversing the cause of the acute situation. [*See* Part Two: "Specific Treatment Modalities," Section A, II. "Guidelines on dialysis."] Further, there is *no* possibility that a viable person will emerge at the other end of the acute situation. In addition, it could be argued that to do useless things to a patient in these circumstances harms the person—even if the person is unconscious. It should be remembered that as a group we believe that persons can even be injured after death—there are strong prohibitions among us against disfiguring corpses.

While it is possible to see the treatment of an episode of disease as an isolated event, and this even facilitates technical decisions, to do so depersonalizes the event as surely as treating merely a body part depersonalizes the part. If peritoneal dialysis (as in Jim Adams's case) is merely considered a device to lower (say) the serum creatinine or the serum potassium, then the future that is being considered is the future of Jim Adams's fluid and electrolyte compartment. But if, as most people would agree, the future of Jim Adams is what is at stake, then dialysis falls from the central position and the person of Jim Adams becomes the key. How will lowering the serum creatinine (or serum potassium) affect the future of Jim Adams? When the goal is the good of a person, it is *always* implied that because of the intervention, the future will be better than an alternative future without the intervention (even if the future holds death). Jim Adams will die with or without dialysis. He will not return to clear-headed consciousness so that he may have more precious hours with friends or family. Nothing about the dialysis promises to improve the future of Jim Adams. But, it might be argued, we do not know what Jim Adams would have said. Perhaps he would have chosen to remain alive on dialysis without there being a real chance of his ever returning to himself. Perhaps the image of continuing and increasing life supports to his failing body would meet his idea of a desirable future.

That does not seem probable. Perhaps no one reading this would believe that that image met *his or her* idea of a good future. Even those who believe, for religious or other reasons, that life support should *always* be continued probably would not like the idea of that future for themselves. We cannot know with certainty what Jim Adams would have wanted—even if he were alive and clear-headed we could not know with certainty whether what he said was what he meant. But we accept the uncertainty that attends people's declarations of self-determination because the alternative—overriding people's autonomous choices for their lives—is worse. All other patients with AIDS have avoided the fate befalling Jim Adams by refusing resuscitative measures should their circumstances be the same. The doctors who are caring for him feel the same way for themselves. Society at large has expressed itself similarly, as countless expositions in the media have shown. In the tradition of medicine, what the doctor or the community believe a patient would want figures importantly in decisionmaking when the patient cannot decide for himself or herself. Not to extend to patients who lack capacity to decide for themselves, such as Jim Adams, our common understanding of what is best for dying sick persons, *denies them membership in the collective human community at the very moment when they need the help of others most.* It is necessary to accept the small uncertainty as to whether Jim Adams would agree with us, in order to avoid the worse alternative of treating him as though he were completely alone. Jim Adams should not be started on dialysis.

7. Was She Ready to Die?
The Case of Grandmother Chang

On a cold snowy day, Dr. Thomas Chang stomped his way across town to visit his grandmother, who was a patient at a hospital. He was in good spirits, as he had learned that she would be discharged in two days. He had wrapped a silken scarf that she had brought from China many years ago for her to wear home and was looking forward to her gentle smile of delight at this.

His grandmother, Ling Chang, who was eighty-four years old, had been admitted to the hospital four days earlier for medical observation, monitoring, and treatment of a condition that was not critical. She had improved and was told that she could soon return home.

As Dr. Chang entered his grandmother's hospital room, she did not turn to greet him. His medical instincts came to the fore, and he noted that she had poor color, no pulse, and wasn't breathing. He realized with a terrible suddenness that she had suffered a cardiac arrest and immediately began CPR. After a few cycles, he ran into the corridor and hailed a nurse. He told her that he was a physician and asked her to call a cardiac code. Seconds later, a staff physician and several nurses rushed into the room and ordered Dr. Chang, who had resumed CPR, to leave.

After he was gone, the physician and nurses administered no further treatment, and Mrs. Chang died. The physician who had responded to the code, Dr. Thompson, told a stunned Dr. Chang afterward that his grandmother had been given a "DNR" status because of her age and debilitated condition, and that he and the nurses, therefore, could not resuscitate her.

Dr. Chang was extremely angry about his grandmother's death. He consulted his lawyer, who recommended that he take the hospital and Dr. Thompson and his team to court. In his complaint, Dr. Chang alleged that the hospital's employees and agents "knowingly, willfully, maliciously, intentionally, recklessly, and without the patient's consent or the consent of a responsible family member, had assigned Mrs. Chang to a 'DNR' status when she was in a non-critical medical condition and improving and that they had refused to perform necessary life-saving procedures."

Should Mrs. Chang have been made a "No Code"? Why did this happen? What do you think should be done at this institution in the future?

Commentary by Ruth Oratz

At present, policies about instituting or withholding cardiopulmonary resuscitation vary greatly among health care institutions. Most patients do not make decisions about resuscitation in advance of cardiopulmonary arrest. Only when arrest is imminent or, indeed, has occurred does anyone ask, "Should this patient be resuscitated?" In some institutions, all patients are subjected to full resuscitative efforts. In others, criteria for who should and should not receive several different versions of resuscitation are carefully spelled out. However, for a great number of patients, decisions about code status are made in an *ad hoc* and arbitrary fashion—based more on the physician's personal biases than on an informed decision by the patient. For the elderly, mentally impaired, physically handicapped, and seriously or terminally ill patient there is often little assurance that any considerations other than the physician's preference will determine resuscitation status.

The case of Mrs. Chang illustrates the pitfalls of the current policy (or lack of policy) for determination of DNR status. Mrs. Chang died in the hospital of a potentially reversible condition because the staff physician apparently decided that she was "too old and debilitated" to be resuscitated. In fact, the patient had been managing quite well at home, was active and mentally intact, and had no major medical problems. She suffered from a minor condition that only required some monitoring in the hospital. In addition, she had a caring, involved, and informed family member who could help if she required assistance after discharge. Mrs. Chang should have been resuscitated. How can future Mrs. Changs be assured of a more rational approach for determining their DNR status?

Decisions about cardiopulmonary resuscitation are not different in process from other health care decisions. [*See* Part Two: "Specific Treatment Modalities," Section B. "Cardiopulmonary resuscitation."] They should be made by competent patients after disclosure of the pertinent medical facts and discussion of relevant issues with health care providers, family members, and significant others. DNR status should reflect the patient's own preferences and values. Written or oral advance directives should be followed. As with any other medical decision, if the patient lacks capacity to decide for himself or herself, an appropriate surrogate, subject to the standards outlined in the *Guidelines* [*see* Part One: "The Decisionmaking Process," II., (3) "Identifying the key decisionmaker," and (4) "Making the decision"], should determine the patient's code status.

The responsible health care professional should initiate a discussion concerning CPR and the option of a DNR status with the patient or surrogate at an appropriate point in the patient's clinical course. It is crucial that discussions about this take place in advance of the emergency situation that arises at the time of arrest. Certainly when there is a reasonably likely chance that cardiopulmonary arrest will occur for a patient, DNR status should be determined while that patient is able to participate in the decisionmaking. Patients who are terminally ill, suffering from severe and irreversible illnesses or disabling conditions, or for whom there is some reason to question the presumption of consent to CPR, should be encouraged to discuss whether they wish to have CPR.

The preferences of patients with capacity should be followed. However, it should not be forgotten that currently competent patients retain the right to revoke a previous directive. If a patient no longer has decisionmaking capacity, advance directives stating the patient's wishes about CPR should be respected. Neither the family nor the physician has the right to override the competent patient's wishes. Even if it is the consensus of well-qualified medical professionals that resuscitation will be ultimately futile, if a competent patient has requested CPR, initial resuscitative efforts should be made. Patients may value the extra days of life that CPR will allow, and their families may need the reassurance that everything possible has been done that such initial attempts provide. "Show codes" or "slow codes" should not be undertaken. There are, however, some limits to the patient's rights to demand CPR. If resuscitation and the subsequent maintenance of life support would be ultimately futile for the patient *and* injurious to other parties (for example, because the patient occupies an ICU bed or ventilator that would be beneficial to another patient), then ethically, CPR and life support may be withheld or withdrawn. If a patient is being considered for CPR after one or more attempts have failed and it is highly unlikely that the patient's downhill course can be reversed, CPR may be discontinued. CPR and other resuscitative and life support measures should not be instituted for patients who are brain dead, except for temporary support of the body while arrangements for organ donation are made.

In general, consent for resuscitation should be presumed when there is no DNR order. Explicit consent should not be required for CPR. There may be some special circumstances in which CPR may be forgone in the absence of a DNR order when patients lack the capacity to decide for themselves and have no readily available surrogate at the time of cardiopulmonary arrest. For example, it might be appropriate not to resuscitate patients who are imminently dying from a known, fatal, and progressive illness with no reversible component or for whom the resuscitative effort would be painful *and* medically futile or merely experimental. It must be emphasized, however, that it is vastly preferable to initiate discussion with such patients early in the course of illness before they become incapacitated or to seek surrogate decisionmaking for incompetent patients. It is important that DNR discussions not occur in the Emergency Room or Intensive Care Unit, when the patient is already extremely debilitated and families and friends are distraught, but in the ambulatory setting when the patient is still capable of making decisions about care.

There may be circumstances in which the presumption in favor of resuscitation should hold until a thorough discussion of the issues with the patient can take place. Examples of such situations might include:(1) A young bride and her new husband are in a car crash following their wedding ceremony and the groom is killed. The bride is seriously wounded and requires emergency intervention. She declares that she, too, wishes to die. In the event of arrest, she should be resuscitated, as it is likely that the circumstances have clouded her judgment. (2) A fifty-year-old man is brought to the hospital with a large anterior wall myocardial infarction (a dangerous heart attack). He is medically unstable, and it is possible that emotional stress might worsen his condition. It is also likely that CPR would be successful if he should suffer a cardiac arrest shortly after admission. He should be resuscitated, if this is needed. (3) A seventy-two-year-old woman is assaulted and raped while walking in the park. She is brought to the Emergency Room unconscious and suffers a respiratory arrest. She, too, should be resuscitated. In these examples, the decision to resuscitate prevails because there is a presumption that the patient consents to medical treatment and wishes to recover and continue living. Resuscitative efforts should be undertaken in order to restore the patient's functional capacity at which time discussion of further treatment should ensue.

Arbitrary criteria such as age, sex, religion, ethnic origin, medical or psychiatric diagnosis, socio-economic status, or ability to work should not determine code status. Patients such as Mrs. Chang should be assured that, as a matter of institutional policy, they will be given the opportunity to determine their own code status or, if this is not possible, that there is a presumption in favor of resuscitating them.

8. The Patient as Stranger: The Case of Mr. Jaworski

Mr. Jaworski was a sixty-nine-year-old man with home addresses in two different states, as he traveled around the country on business a great deal. He was divorced and had two daughters, but he had not been in touch with his former wife or children for years. Mr. Jaworski had coronary artery disease for which he had received a bypass graft eight years ago. He also had a history of melena (blood in the feces), anemia, weight loss, atrial fibrillation (irregular heart beat), and two prior cardiac arrests.

Mr. Jaworski entered the hospital in a state in which he did not have a home address with a history of two hours of substernal chest pain. He was admitted to the Coronary Care Unit to rule out a myocardial infarction. On admission to the CCU he told the attending physician, resident, and nurse that he did not wish to be resuscitated should his heart arrest and said that he had expressed his preferences earlier in a hospital in another state and in a "Living Will" in yet a third state. Staff members did not know Mr. Jaworski and did not have copies of his previous records or "Living Will." They were uneasy about not resuscitating him. They expressed uncertainty about whether his previous written and oral statements had legal effect in this state and decided that therefore they could not classify him as a "No Code."

When Mr. Jaworski had a cardiac arrest seven hours later, he received full cardiopulmonary resuscitation. Following this, he was unresponsive, in decorticate position (hands and feet curled up in position indicating major neurological damage), and dependent on the respirator for breathing. He was also noted to have convulsive activity of his left cheek and tongue.

Mr. Jaworski's attending physician, resident, and nurse met again to discuss his current condition and their earlier conversations with him. At this time, they decided that it would be appropriate to make him a "No Code." A DNR order was written, and Mr. Jaworski died three days later, after he had a second arrest, without ever regaining consciousness.

Should Mr. Jaworski have been resuscitated when he had his first cardiac arrest in this hospital? Should he have been resuscitated when he had his second cardiac arrest? What effect, if any, should the statements that he made on admission have had on his treatment?

Commentary by David H. Miller

Who is ultimately responsible for determining when it is appropriate not to perform cardiopulmonary resuscitation—the patient or the physician? This is the basic ethical dilemma presented by the case of Mr. Jaworski. He has known ischemic heart disease, has undergone coronary artery bypass surgery, has survived two previous cardiac arrests, has presenting symptoms suggestive of an acute myocardial infarction with inherent risks of life-threatening complications, and requests that his newly appointed physicians not resuscitate him in the event of cardiac arrest. His history is complicated by the clinical evidence for the presence of some other (as yet undiagnosed) ongoing disease manifesting as melena, anemia, and weight loss which could represent anything from a benign to a malignant process.

Success in unraveling the components of this ethical dilemma depends upon the thorough evaluation of the decisionmaking process. Fundamental to this process is the need to establish with as much certainty as possible the nature and extent of the underlying medical conditions, the possible therapeutic options, and the projected outcome with specific forms of therapy. Details about the severity of Mr. Jaworski's cardiac disease, its impact on his functional status, and the range of therapies offered, including their potential risks and benefits, are not provided. However, knowledge about these matters is essential to insuring that Mr. Jaworski's decision is an informed one.

So, too, must Mr. Jaworski have the capacity to make the decision at hand: he must be able to comprehend the choices involved, he must be able to select from among them, and he must be able to take responsibility for his final choice.

Uncertainties about any of these components of the decisionmaking process can lead to the questioning of the appropriateness of the final decision about cardiopulmonary resuscitation, irrespective of who makes it. For instance, disagreement might arise over the interpretation of Mr. Jaworski's functional status. Permanent impairment resulting from the prior cardiac arrests might be viewed as intolerable by the patient and inconsequential by the physicians. Similarly, the potential threat of an existing colon cancer might be devastating news to the patient but only evidence supporting the need for additional diagnostic studies to the physicians. Or, analgesic drugs administered in the Emergency Room might be considered anxiety-relieving agents which enhance decisionmaking capacity by the patient and mind-altering agents which impair decisionmaking capacity by the physician.

The extent of the underlying disease and the potential reversibility of a life-threatening event influence the judgment about the potential value of cardiopulmonary resuscitation. As the severity of the underlying disease increases and the likelihood of successful resuscitation diminishes, the case for initiating resuscitation becomes less compelling.

Just as uncertainty may exist about the underlying clinical condition, so too may misunderstanding develop about the nature and implications of resuscitation itself. It may be distinguished from other forms of treatment, in particular, because of its need for immediate initiation, its multi-faceted components (which may include chest compressions, electrical cardioversions, intubation with respirator support, and drug infusions), and its unpredictable outcome (varying from death to functional impairment to full recovery). In addition, the fundamental presumption in favor of providing life-saving treatment, rather than denying it, necessitates that resuscitation be initiated unless otherwise specified. As a result, consent must be obtained to withhold cardiopulmonary resuscitation rather than to undertake it.

Since patients cannot participate in deliberations about the use of cardiopulmonary resuscitation after a cardiac arrest has occurred, decisionmaking must be done in advance of and in anticipation of an acute life-threatening event and is subject to the inherent difficulties in solving hypothetical, rather than actual, problems. This raises the possibility that decisions made in the pre-arrest setting do not pertain to the event itself and that unanticipated circumstances might direct therapy along a course contrary to the patient's previously expressed wishes.

Decisionmaking when a patient has lost the capacity to decide requires the identification of a surrogate to act on the patient's behalf. This person, often the patient's spouse, may naturally assume the role. However, when no such person has been identified, as in the case of Mr. Jaworski, an alternate person must be selected, ideally by the patient. The need for this is especially crucial when the patient chooses an individual who is not a naturally appearing surrogate, as is the next of kin. The failure of Mr. Jaworski to identify such a person in advance of his cardiac arrest placed the burden of decisionmaking on the staff without the benefit of surrogate oversight after the resuscitation effort left the patient in an unresponsive state.

An understanding of the issues involved in determining resuscitation status helps to resolve the conflict between the patient's demand that the procedure not be performed and the physician's insistence upon performing it. The ethical principle of autonomy, that patients have ultimate control over what happens to their bodies, is tested against the principle of beneficence, that experienced physicians must do what is immediately good for their patients. In fact, there is evidence to suggest that the criteria of informed decisionmaking and intact decisionmaking capacity have been met in this case.

Mr. Jaworski experienced the manifestations of ischemic heart disease for several years, during which he had two cardiac arrests. He presumably had a thorough understanding of the nature of the disease processes and potential outcomes. One might argue that he was even better qualified to judge the potential benefits and risks of resuscitation than most (if not all) physicians. Although the cause of the gastrointestinal bleeding was not determined, its importance as a factor in deciding resuscitation status seems small compared with the extensive cardiac history.

Moreover, there was no evidence to suggest that Mr. Jaworski lacked decisionmaking capacity—indeed, his decisions appeared to be not only well thought out, but well documented with a Living Will and records from previous hospitalizations. The uncertainty about the legal authority of these documents should not have been used as a means to negate the expressed wishes of the patient. Similarly, the physicians' and nurses' unfamiliarity with the patient himself should not have precluded acceptance of his directives about subsequent therapies. Mr. Jaworski's wishes not to be resuscitated should have prevailed at the outset, and no resuscitation effort should have been initiated. It follows that the decision not to resuscitate him after his first resuscitation in this hospital was appropriate.

The *Guidelines* provide a clear template for resolving these kinds of problems in Part One: "The Decisionmaking Process." They stipulate the need to determine as objectively as possible the underlying disease processes, the expected prognoses, and the potential risks and benefits of therapeutic interventions. Such determinations could have clarified any uncertainties about the patient's and the physicians' understanding of the medical aspects of this case.

The *Guidelines* establish the need for the assessment and determination of patient decisionmaking capacity and provide procedures for patient management when capacity is lacking. [*See* Part One, II., (c) "Identifying the key decisionmaker."] The *Guidelines* stipulate the need for the patient to identify a surrogate decisionmaker before the patient's decisionmaking capacity is impaired. [*See* Part Three: "Prospective Planning, Guidelines on Advance Directives."] This would have created the protective mechanism for third-party oversight of the patient's care after the cardiac arrest.

Finally, the *Guidelines* support the importance and necessity of ascertaining patient's wishes about therapeutic interventions upon themselves and creating a mechanism for ensuring that their wishes are respected.

9. "I've Lived Long Enough": The Case of Sarah Green

Two years ago, Sarah Green, now aged ninety-one, had left her apartment to buy some food for dinner at a neighborhood store. Walking was not easy for her, as she had arthritis and osteoporosis, so she took a short-cut through an alley next to her apartment. As she entered the alley, she was jumped by two men who pushed her roughly to the ground and ran off with her purse.

A neighbor found Mrs. Green soon after and called an ambulance that took her to a nearby hospital. In the Emergency Room, she was diagnosed as having a broken hip, and she was sent to surgery to have it repaired. A week later, Mrs. Green was transferred from the hospital to Goldengrove Nursing Home, since she lived alone and had no one to take care of her. Mrs. Green had been widowed six years earlier and her son had been killed in Vietnam. Her only living relative is a niece with whom she is not close.

Since her admission to Goldengrove, her general condition has slowly declined. She is very frail, but can walk with help. Her major functional disability is a progressive loss of vision, which she finds very distressing, as her favorite pastime is reading. For a while, friends from her old neighborhood came by to read to her, but she no longer has visitors.

Six months ago, Mrs. Green was diagnosed as suffering from a preleukemic blood condition that required regular blood transfusions every month. This therapy was promptly begun, and her condition has stabilized. Her future prognosis is good if she continues the transfusions. The transfusions leave her feeling "washed out" for a day, but she has no other pain or difficulty with them. Even so, Mrs. Green has informed the doctor and nurses several times that she no longer wants the transfusions. She has also told others that she is ready to die. Her niece, who has been contacted, supports her aunt in her decision.

A psychiatrist has interviewed Mrs. Green extensively about her desire to forgo the transfusions. Mrs. Green has told her psychiatrist exactly what she told the others—that she has lived long enough, that she is no longer contributing anything to the world, and that since she no longer can have the enjoyment of reading, there is no point in her continuing to live. Although Mrs. Green occasionally exhibits lapses of short-term memory, the psychiatrist has found that she has decision making capacity and that she can understand her situation.

Each month when the nurses administer the transfusion, Mrs. Green protests, but eventually they persuade her, and she submits to the procedure. Should they continue to coax her to have transfusions?

Commentary by Paul Homer and Harry R. Moody

The nursing and medical staff caring for Mrs. Green are understandably and appropriately troubled by her request to have monthly blood transfusions for a pre-leukemic condition terminated. From a medical point of view, her disease is treatable with regular transfusions and her prognosis is good. Mrs. Green, however, has a dim view of her prognosis. Her objection to further treatment appears to be based on a personal assessment of the quality of life the transfusions make possible. The central issue in this case is how the conflict between Mrs. Green's "medical" prognosis and her own view of her prognosis should be resolved.

The ethical principle of self-determination (also referred to as the principle of autonomy or respect for persons) holds that a competent individual ought to be free to make decisions in accordance with his or her values, purposes, and preferences. Since these are relevant considerations, medical indications are not sufficient grounds for decisions regarding treatment. A medical prognosis represents only one factor among many that the decisionmaker must consider. The principle of self-determination puts the competent individual in the position of primary arbiter of all these factors. In this case, a psychiatrist has determined that Mrs. Green is fully competent and capable of understanding her situation. Therefore, Mrs. Green has at least a *prima facie* right to refuse further blood transfusions. Her caregivers have a correlative duty to respect her choice.

Although the principle of self-determination supports the right to refuse life-saving medical treatment, some may argue that the case of Mrs. Green raises separate issues because it involves an attempt to commit suicide. She knows that the consequence of refusing treatment is death, and yet continues to refuse it. Surely she wants to die and must be considered suicidal. However, it would be misleading to construe Mrs. Green's request as an act of suicide. Suicide is a very difficult concept to define. For instance, we usually regard the depressed but otherwise healthy and recovering patient who jumps to his death as a case of suicide. On the other hand, we do not ordinarily view a refusal of chemotherapy by an individual with terminal and irreversible cancer as falling into the same category. Between these two extremes lies a range of cases that are much more difficult to classify. The case of Mrs. Green is one such example.

A key element in any definition of suicide is intentionality. A person can knowingly engage in a host of risk-filled activities that could result in death, without attempting suicide. Suicide assumes a clear intention on the part of the agent to terminate his or her life. One can forgo treatment, foreseeing that death is likely, without necessarily intending to bring about death. For Mrs. Green, the intention is ambiguous. She has informed others she is *"ready* to die" and that "there is no point in continuing to live." These statements are not conclusive evidence of an intention to terminate life. Moreover, her actions do not seem to support the claim that she has a clear intention to terminate her life.

However, we are still left with the question, "Is her refusal morally justified?" Any attempt to answer this question should begin by recognizing that medical treatments invariably impose burdens at the same time that they attempt to provide benefits. The burdens can take many forms—such as physical, psychological, or financial—and can vary in degree. The difficulty lies in weighing the benefits and burdens, that is, in determining an acceptable balance. Some treatments are clearly inappropriate for certain patients because the benefits are likely to be negligible while the burdens are great—for example, surgery and chemotherapy for a patient with end-stage metastatic cancer. However, trying to determine what to do when the benefits and burdens appear balanced is a more vexing task.

In Mrs. Green's case, her health care team believes that the transfusions provide great benefit—prolonged life—without being overly burdensome. But there are burdens: they include subjection to an invasive procedure and the small risk of infection and other complications, especially for an older person. Perhaps a greater burden is the psychological toll that the need for chronic transfusions can exact. Many people might accept these burdens gladly in light of the benefits provided. But that does not answer the question, "Do the benefits outweigh the burdens *for Mrs. Green?"* Benefits and burdens of treatments are borne by the patient, and their value and disvalue to a patient's life are best understood by that patient. That is why competent persons are granted the *prima facie* right to make decisions regarding medical treatment. In this case, the burdens of the blood transfusions for Mrs. Green's life can and should be determined by Mrs. Green. Despite Mrs. Green's *prima facie* right to refuse blood transfusions, each month the nursing staff "persuades" her to accept the treatment. In addressing the conditions in which a competent patient's refusal of treatment can be justifiably denied, Tom Beauchamp and James Childress have argued, "A refusal of treatment in life-threatening circumstances may be overridden if and only if nontreatment would produce or would be reasonably expected to produce significant harm to others or violate the rights of others."[1] The burden of proof that one of these overriding conditions is met falls on those persons who wish to override this right.

In the case of Mrs. Green, it is difficult to see how others would be significantly harmed or how their rights would be violated by respecting her refusal. The health care staff could claim that their moral or professional duty would be violated by allowing Mrs. Green to forgo blood transfusions that provide some benefit. But even if this point is valid, it is doubtful whether it provides sufficient grounds to override Mrs. Green's right to refuse treatment.

The nursing and medical staff are appropriately troubled by Mrs. Green's decision. The health care professional's sense of moral obligation to care for patients, especially those who feel that life is not worth living, remains important. Stanley Hauerwas has been a critic of society's readiness to embrace notions of a right to commit suicide, and more generally, a right to die. He argues that these notions may represent the "final affirmation and sealing of a long process of abandonment by the community" and that "we may have unwittingly affirmed a society that no longer wishes to provide the conditions for the miracle of trust and community."[2] Hauerwas's critique may be disputed, but he rightly suggests reasons for concern about an all-too-accommodating recognition of the right to die.

Mrs. Green seems to be an excellent candidate for this type of concern. Although the "persuasion" used each month by the nursing staff is not described in any detail, it is conceivable that it expresses care, compassion, and trust. The staff, however, should explore ways to sustain that care, rather than muddling through from month to month. Perhaps with creative social service planning, the institution and staff could provide a more stimulating environment for Mrs. Green. Volunteer visits and the use of books-on-tape might improve her outlook.

Expressions of care also encompass respecting a patient's thoughtful decisions concerning treatment. Efforts to improve Mrs. Green's quality of life do not obviate the need of caregivers to acknowledge her right to refuse the blood tranfusions. The staff's persuasion is efficacious each month, but that "she *submits* to the procedure" raises serious doubts about the consensual basis of the treatment. Is there substantial coercion involved here? There is an undeniable element of paternalism involved in the month-by-month "persuasion" that finally results in the transfusions. This paternalism is of the most extreme kind: refusing to acquiesce to a competent patient's right to choose in the name of that patient's own benefit. Paternalism of that kind is contrary to professional, legal, and moral traditions.

Mrs. Green raises painful questions about her life in Goldengrove that should not be ignored. A process of open and extended discussion between Mrs. Green and her caregivers must commence. They should talk about Mrs. Green's view of her life and her likely death if transfusions cease. The health care team should explore with Mrs. Green strategies for improving her quality of life, and Mrs. Green should be asked to articulate the exact nature of her protest against the transfusions. An explanation ought to be sought as to why her spoken preferences seem to contradict her actual behavior. Only subsequent to this discussion can both parties feel satisfied that a morally responsible decision has been reached.

The *Guidelines* that bear most directly on the case of Mrs. Green can be found in Part One: "Making Treatment Decisions." Here the view that competent patients have a *prima facie* right to forgo any life-sustaining treatment is presented. Mrs. Green is a competent patient with a severe and irreversible illness. The right to decide belongs to her. In addition, Part Two: "Specific Treatment Modalities," Section B. "Treatment for life-threatening bleeding" recommends that professionals initiate discussions about forgoing treatment for bleeding when there is some reason to question the presumption of the patient's consent. Although Mrs. Green is not in an emergency situation, the recommendation to discuss these decisions with her would still apply.

A competent patient will consider his or her decision within the context of a relationship with health care professionals and with the benefit of their expertise. It is critical to underscore the importance of talking things over. [*See* Part One: "Making Treatment Decisions," II., (2) "Evaluation and discussion," (b) "Facilitating discussion."] The discussion alluded to in the case description would seem to amount to little more than crisis intervention. Mrs. Green and the staff should discuss the blood transfusions after the crisis has passed in order to facilitate careful deliberation. Mrs. Green also should be encouraged to formulate an advance directive indicating her treatment and/or proxy preferences. [*See* Part Three: "Prospective Planning, Guidelines on Advance Directives."] If the decision reached is to terminate the blood transfusions, then other forms of care must be discussed. The health care professionals in this case have a duty to provide at least supportive care in such circumstances. [*See* Part One, II., (6) "Implementing the decision," (b) "Supportive care."]

If the health care team or institution cannot abide by a decision of Mrs. Green to forgo the transfusions, then they should act in accordance with the requirements set out in Part One: II., (8), (e) "Withdrawal of health care professional or institution." This will include notification of Mrs. Green and probably her niece. Transfer to another team or institution should be arranged. If transfer is impossible or if Mrs. Green otherwise wishes to challenge the nursing home's decision, and an institutional ethics committee cannot resolve the matter, legal adjudication may be required.

Finally, Part Six: "Special Problems" includes a pertinent discussion on "Terminating treatment, active voluntary euthanasia, and assisting suicide" in Section I, where relevant conceptual and moral distinctions are formulated.

NOTES

1. Tom L. Beauchamp and James F. Childers, *Principles of Biomedical Ethics*, 2d ed. (New York: Oxford University Press, 1983), p. 90.

2. Stanley Hauerwas, *Truthfulness and Tragedy* (Notre Dame, IN: University of Notre Dame Press, 1977), p. 113.

10. Life Versus Religious Liberty: The Case of Jamal Burke

Jamal Burke, a twenty-six-year-old lawyer, was admitted to the hospital with a history of bloody diarrhea for two weeks. He had lost eight pounds during that time and appeared thin and weak. Except for abdominal tenderness, the physical findings were essentially negative. His hematocrit was 16, and his hemoglobin 4.4 gm. He was diagnosed as having toxic megacolon (dead bowel), and was scheduled for an immediate colectomy (surgical removal of large bowel), as his condition was life-threatening.

When his anesthesiologist came to visit him to discuss the options for anesthesia, Mr. Burke stated that he was a member of the Jehovah's Witness faith and that he did not wish to receive any blood transfusions during surgery. His wife cited a passage from Leviticus 17:10-14 to explain their religion's prohibition against accepting blood. It read: "And whatsoever man there be of the house of Israel, or of the strangers that sojourn among you, that eateth any manner of blood; I will even set my face against that soul that eateth blood, and will cut him off from among his people." Mr. Burke said that he did want surgery since he did not want to die; however, he could not accept blood transfusions during surgery.

The anesthesiologist called Mr. Burke's surgeon. They conferred and disagreed about what should be done. The anesthesiologist believed that Mr. Burke had a right to refuse treatment on the basis of his religious beliefs, even at the risk of death. She said that she would not give Mr. Burke blood transfusions during surgery against his wishes. The surgeon thought that he, as a physician, had an obligation to do everything possible to keep his patients alive and that it would be wrong to stand by and watch a preventable death. They agreed to try to resolve the problem by talking to Mr. Burke to see if they could get him to change his mind about receiving blood transfusions.

The two physicians told Mr. Burke that they hoped he would reconsider his decision so that they could treat him at their hospital. They explained that the institution had a written policy that required the administration of life-sustaining blood transfusions to all patients, regardless of the wishes of those who were Jehovah's Witnesses. Although the institution acknowledged the right of patients to refuse blood, it maintained that this right does not extend to the point of allowing patients to die for want of life-saving blood transfusions. Patients who did not accept this policy were free to go to another hospital.

Mr. Burke suggested to the physicians that he was at a lower risk of death if they operated on him without giving him blood transfusions than if they discharged him to another hospital, for he might not survive the transfer. In addition, he said that he would rather take his chances on surgery without blood transfusions at this hospital because of its excellent reputation, rather than at another. Mr. Burke also said that he or his wife would file a legal complaint against them if they refused to respect his decision. He claimed that the surgeon should have told him about the policy of the hospital when he first arrived and that it was now too late for them to discharge him.

Should Mr. Burke be operated upon in the hospital to which he has been admitted? If so, should he receive blood transfusions during surgery? If not, what alternatives should be made available to him?

Commentary by Susan M. Wolf

This case raises two main questions: what decisionmaking procedures should be followed when a patient wishes to refuse transfusion on religious grounds, and how should conflict be resolved between the patient's refusal and a hospital's policy requiring transfusion, as well as a physician's objection to participating in allowing a patient to forgo transfusions?

Patients with decisionmaking capacity have the moral and legal right to refuse life-sustaining treatment, including life-saving transfusion. When patients refuse treatment on nonreligious grounds, their moral right to refuse rests on the value of self-determination or autonomy. Indeed, that value demands respect for a patient's decision even when idiosyncratic; if a person in exercising his autonomy had to decide as everyone else would, there effectively would be no right to self-determination. The legal right to refuse life-sustaining treatment rests on two bases: the right in common law to be free of nonconsensual bodily invasion and the constitutional right to privacy. Although the courts have discussed countervailing state interests that might outweigh the individual's right, those interests have rarely been considered to prevail.

When the patient refuses treatment on religious grounds, the moral and legal basis for his right to refuse is additionally bolstered by the fact that he is asserting a right to religious freedom. Indeed, the courts have recognized the right of Jehovah's Witnesses to refuse life-sustaining transfusions, at least when the patient is an adult with no dependent children, as in the case of Jamal Burke.

The process of making a decision about whether to forgo transfusions when the patient is a Jehovah's Witness should consequently follow the same basic format as when a patient wishes to refuse treatment on other grounds. There are, however, several changes required in the process. Two are relevant in this case. First, the responsible health care professional should speak with the patient outside the presence of family members or clergy. Because the right to refuse treatment is a right to self-determination, it is important to ascertain whether the patient's decision is his own, free of duress. Sometimes family or clergy of the same faith will pressure the patient to refuse transfusion, when the patient may be ambivalent or may not really want to forgo treatment at all. In the Burke case, it would be advisable to speak to Mr. Burke outside of his wife's presence.

Second, whenever there are indications that a patient is a Jehovah's Witness—and so may wish to forgo transfusion—health care professionals should promptly ascertain the patient's wishes and resolve the question of whether the patient will be transfused. If a Jehovah's Witness wishes to forgo transfusions, that must be determined in advance of a bleeding crisis, lest the patient be transfused and his right to refuse be lost. Early attention to the issue also allows the physicians to explore whether alternatives to the use of blood or blood products are feasible. In this case, the matter first arose when the anesthesiologist met with the patient before surgery. Ideally, the matter should be dealt with as early as possible.

The other major problem in this case is the conflict between Mr. Burke's right to refuse transfusion and the surgeon's and hospital's positions. An institution should consider long and hard before it creates a policy that some form of treatment cannot be forgone within its walls. Patients have the right to refuse treatment. To force patients to surrender that right in order to receive the care that the institution offers is a drastic step. This case shows that indeed at least one physician practicing within that institution is in fact willing to care for a Jehovah's Witness refusing transfusion. A better policy might be to establish a list of those surgeons, anesthesiologists, and other health care professionals willing to care for Jehovah's Witnesses refusing transfusion. Such a policy could also create procedures to help identify early those patients refusing transfusion. Then if a health care professional caring for the patient concludes he or she cannot honor the patient's wishes, the professional and patient can pursue the option of transferring the patient's care to a professional on the list.

Here, however, the institution already has a policy blocking refusal of transfusion altogether. Yet Mr. Burke was given no notice of that policy before or at the time of admission. He had no opportunity at that juncture to consider whether to enter another institution that would honor his preference.

Mr. Burke is correct that patients should receive notice of such a policy at arrival.

At this point, the institution and its physicians have undertaken his care and cannot abandon him. Having given the patient no notice that he surrenders certain rights at the door, they cannot now force him to do so. This is particularly the case if, as Mr. Burke suggests, transfer poses serious risk to the patient's health. Institutions, however, should make every effort to respect a health care professional's conscientious objection to participating in Mr. Burke's chosen course of treatment. The institution should assist in finding another surgeon who is willing to operate without transfusing the patient.

The *Guidelines* are in accord with this resolution. Part Two, "Specific Treatment Modalities," Section B, "Treatment for life-threatening bleeding," states that the right of Jehovah's Witnesses to refuse life-saving blood transfusions should be respected. That section urges health care professionals to confer with such patients as early as possible to establish whether the patient will be transfused if life-threatening bleeding occurs. It also counsels health care providers to speak to the patient alone to make sure the patient is refusing transfusion of his own free will.

Section (8), (d), "Disagreement on the health care team," and (e) "Withdrawal of health care professional or institution" deals with objections by a health care institution or individual professionals to honoring a patient's refusal of transfusion. In keeping with the case analysis above, that section recommends that an institution establish a list of those professionals willing to care for a Jehovah's Witness patient refusing transfusion. That subsection together with the corresponding section of the "Guidelines on the decisionmaking process" in Part One [Part One, II., (8), (d) and (e)] also recommend that a health care professional's conscientious objection to caring for a patient refusing transfusion be honored. The objecting professional, with the patient's or surrogate's consent, may transfer the patient's care to another professional willing to care for the patient and to honor the request.

11. Too Sick to Eat:
The Case of Joseph

Five years ago, Joseph Davies, a seventy-five-year-old bachelor, began to forget people's names and where he had put things. Before this, he had been quite sharp. He also began to have difficulties with his daily activities and in attending to his personal needs. Joseph lived with his brother, Lester, and Lester's wife. The brothers had always been close, and Lester and his wife were pleased to be able to help him. However, after a while they found it increasingly difficult to provide the degree of care that Joseph needed.

One day when Lester was feeding him, Joseph choked on his food and went into respiratory distress. Lester's wife immediately telephoned 911, and Joseph was rushed to a hospital. There he was treated for aspiration pneumonia, and a nasogastric tube was inserted to feed him. The tube was removed after five days, as Joseph seemed miserable with it. The hospital social worker strongly recommended nursing home placement for Joseph, and after talking this over with their religious counselor, Lester and his wife decided that this would be best.

At the nursing home, Joseph continued to have difficulty in swallowing and showed no interest in eating. The nursing staff told Lester that a nasogastric tube would have to be inserted once again, as Joseph could not be adequately nourished by oral feedings. Lester reluctantly agreed to this.

Joseph withdrew to a point where he seemed generally oblivious to his surroundings and to other people. He no longer spoke and had no control of his basic bodily functions. He remained in bed in a semi-fetal position. He could move in bed to a moderate extent and responded to painful stimuli. His primary physician told Lester that Joseph was in a severe state of senile dementia.

Four months after the nasogastric tube was reinserted, Lester requested that it be removed. He said that it was prolonging Joseph's life unreasonably and was very uncomfortable. He and his wife had spoken about the matter with their religious counselor again, and they had agreed that they did not want Joseph to suffer any longer from such extraordinary means. They believed that he had reached "a time to die" spoken of in Ecclesiastes.

Joseph's physician removed his feeding tube and ordered him placed on "supportive care only." When the nursing staff began to feed him by inserting liquified food into his mouth with a syringe, Lester became very upset because Joseph choked. He requested that Joseph be fed only with a cup and spoon. This was done. Joseph was sedated, kept comfortable, and offered food and water by cup and spoon. He died a few weeks later.

Should the medical and nursing staff have followed Lester's instructions and removed the nasogastric tube from Joseph?

Commentary by Daniel Callahan

The case of Joseph is a perplexing one for a number of reasons. We do not know what Joseph himself might have thought about someone in his state. We have no clues, and neither apparently does his brother, about Joseph's values in situations of this kind. Even if we did know, say, that Joseph would not have wanted his life extended by aggressive medical intervention, we might still have trouble deciding whether tube-feeding should count as "medical" treatment. Even if, moreover, we knew that Joseph would not have wanted tube-feeding, it would not be immediately evident that we would have the right to honor such a request. Joseph was not dying from his advanced and severe dementia. One might argue that it would be the removal of the tube that would kill him, not his underlying disease.

I mention all of these reasons for hesitation and doubt to indicate how sorely decisions about stopping nutrition test our understanding of the termination of treatment. While many people give some prior thought to the possibility that they might want their medical treatment stopped, they do not always and automatically encompass the medical provision of nutrition within the scope of such a choice. Medical professionals who might readily be prepared to stop obvious medical treatment often feel differently about cessation of nutrition. This uncertainty is not hard to understand. Both long-standing custom and the natural instincts of most people lead them to feed other people, whatever their physical condition; and certainly this has been the case from time immemorial in medicine. Food and water have not been thought of as "treatment." They are simply what we all need, sick or well, to survive.

Yet the advances of medical technology in keeping people alive, making it possible now not only to provide nutrition through a simple nasogastric tube, but intravenously or through a line into the stomach, change both the meaning of feeding someone and the meaning of a medical intervention. One common view emphasizes the provision of nutrition as the key moral item; the method, whether simple or not, technological or not, is irrelevant.

To fail to provide nutrition is thus to fail the most basic ethic of medicine, that of caring. Another view emphasizes the way in which the nutrition is provided, and the fact that it is provided artificially—that is, by an artifact, not by hand—becomes the crucial moral factor. Under the former view, the cessation of nutrition would always be wrong, the violation of a fundamental rule of medical ethics. Under the latter view, if it would be acceptable to stop medical treatment, it would be equally acceptable to stop artificially-provided nutrition, especially when the feeding itself increases the pain and suffering.

It should be noted that I have not mentioned the fact of Joseph's severe dementia. What is its moral relevance in this circumstance, one in which we have no instructions from the patient himself about what should done in such a case? Joseph, though severely impaired, is still a living human being, and although he is on an irreversibly downhill course he is not imminently dying. There is every reason, then, to give the continuance of life the benefit of the doubt. Were it not for the perception that the feeding seemed to increase Joseph's misery, there would be no strong grounds to stop it. But the burden of the feeding does have moral significance. We might decide we had no obligation to impose upon a patient a course of caring, whether we call it treatment or not, which causes pain without relieving or reversing the underlying cause of the illness.

But is it not the case that the cessation of nutrition will itself be the cause of death, and thus in effect a form of direct euthanasia? I do not believe that is so in this kind of case. It is the disease that, apparently, has a role in making him choke on food provided orally, and the same condition that makes him "miserable" from nasogastric feeding. Were it not for the artificial feeding, nature would have taken his life; his medical care has done nothing but stand in the way of that process. To stop feeding him—particularly when to feed him increases his suffering—is not to kill, but to let his underlying inability to be fed naturally gain the upper hand. The question is whether, in this case, there is an obligation to oppose the physiological deprivations caused by the underlying disease. If unopposed, those deprivations will be the cause of death. Are those, then, who allow that cause to proceed in an unimpeded way morally culpable? I think not. The disease is irreversible, and the tube feeding apparently painful (or so the brother believes). I would find it hard in that circumstance to describe the removal of the tube as a form of culpable direct killing, even though the immediate cause of death will be the lack of nutrition. Death need not be resisted in these circumstances; hence, culpability is absent.

In a situation of this kind, the *Guidelines* would permit the cessation of tube feeding. The brother, acting as surrogate, might come to the reasonable conclusion that, because of the severe (and irreversible) dementia "the patient's life is largely devoid of opportunities to achieve satisfaction," and also that it is "full of pain or suffering with no corresponding benefits." [*See* Part One: "Making Treatment Decisions," II., (4) "Making the decision," (c)

"The patient who lacks decisionmaking capacity," (ii) "The patient who has an illness or disabling condition that is severe and irreversible."] If the pain were absent, then the decision might be more difficult; it would not be utterly clear what a reasonable person might want. In a case of that kind, I would hesitate. We cannot know what, if anything, might be going through the patient's mind; we should, therefore, incline toward the preservation of life. But where there is evidence, or a reasonable belief, that pain or discomfort exists, cessation of tube feeding would seem a decision that a reasonable person could reach. We are then acting for the benefit of the patient.

The presumption of the *Guidelines* is that there is no inherent moral difference between the termination of medical treatment and the termination of artificial feeding. [*See* Part Two: "Specific Treatment Modalities," Section C. "Medical procedures for supplying nutrition and hydration," I. "Introduction."] The *Guidelines* also note, however, the different psychological responses to the two classes of actions. There is a basis for that perception, namely the settled and general conviction of most people that feeding is a basic act of human caring, not a medical act as ordinarily understood. They believe it to be a good thing to do, and our culture has cultivated that belief.

There is a very fine line to be walked here, and it seems to me wrong to be insensitive to that belief or to forcefully override it unless absolutely necessary (and painfully tube-feeding a patient would be such a case). It is a socially tutored conviction that is, on the whole, extraordinarily helpful in reinforcing desirable impulses toward care and nurture. If there is reason to fear that some patients might be artificially fed in ways harmful to their comfort or to their right of self-determination—and there surely is—there are also grounds to be wary of a too-ready acceptance of a cessation of artificial feeding. As a widespread, routine action it could be a symptom of callousness, the suppression by thoughtless routinization of the social instinct to care for others. To support it in individual cases after struggle and thought is acceptable, as in the case of Joseph. To welcome it as a routine is less desirable. The human capacity for self-interested indifference to the lives of others should never be underestimated.

12. "No Patient of Mine Will Ever Starve to Death!" The Case of Mrs. Franklin

One golden fall day, Mrs. Franklin, a sixty-eight-year-old widow, was outside her house raking leaves when she suddenly collapsed on the front lawn. Two of her neighbors ran over to help her, but she did not move or respond in answer to their frantic inquiries. They summoned an ambulance to take her to the hospital and called her two daughters, who arrived at the hospital shortly after she did.

The Emergency Room physician told her daughters that she had suffered a stroke and was comatose. Mrs. Franklin enjoyed a warm relationship with her daughters, and they were determined that she would want for nothing to assist her recovery. After two weeks, however, her physician told them that there was nothing more that the hospital could do for their mother, and she was transferred to Fair View, a large nursing home.

Mrs. Franklin's daughters were very much encouraged when she returned to a semi-conscious state and responded to stimuli a week after her admission. However, she suffered another stroke three months later and again became comatose. She remained in this condition for two years. During that time, the nursing staff maintained her in excellent physical condition. She had no skin breakdown and was hydrated, nourished, and medicated through a nasogastric tube. The tube did not appear to be uncomfortable. Her daughters visited her daily and were very much involved in her care. The older of the two was made legal guardian of Mrs. Franklin's person and property. Gradually, however, neighbors and friends stopped visiting. Her closest friend and neighbor told her daughters, "She is already dead."

At the end of two years, the daughters began to reconsider their decision to provide every available medical measure for their mother. She had once told them that if she were ever in the autumn of her life and in a condition like Karen Quinlan she would not want to be kept alive by medical means. They began to believe that she was in such a condition and that she would no longer want her life prolonged by medical treatment. Both daughters, consequently, signed a written request that artificial nutrition and hydration be ended for their mother. Mrs. Franklin's primary physician concurred with this request.

The request was reviewed by a multidisciplinary patient care committee, as well as by two outside physicians, in accordance with protocol that had been established at Fair View. There was medical agreement that Mrs. Franklin was in a persistent vegetative state and that there was no reasonable probability that she would ever recover. The committee advised that in these circumstances, it was in keeping with the general orientation at Fair View to consider tube feedings "disproportionately burdensome" for Mrs. Franklin. Her physician wrote an order to remove the nasogastric tube and to provide continuing supportive nursing care for her.

The primary nurse who had cared for Mrs. Franklin over the past two years, however, strongly objected to this order. She believed that it was wrong to deny any person food and water, regardless of the hopelessness of his or her condition. "No patient of mine will ever starve to death!" she declared. When Mrs. Franklin's primary physician said he would remove the tube himself, the nurse stated that she would refuse to care for Mrs. Franklin if this were done, as she could not provide normal nursing care to a patent "who was being starved to death."

Should Mrs. Franklin's nasogastric tube be removed? What should be done about the nurse who refuses to care for Mrs. Franklin if the tube is removed?

Commentary by Lois K. Evans

Of primary concern in this case, although by no means the only dilemma raised, is whether the withdrawal of nutrition and hydration is morally justifiable. Issues related to the ethical integrity of health care professionals, decisionmaking authority, and the moral obligations of the institution to patients and employees are also important.

The difficulties inherent in any discussion related to the provision or termination of nutrition and hydration are compounded by the symbolic and emotional significance attributed to food and water. Nourishment and hydration are viewed as basic to life itself and have many social, familial, and religious attachments. Some argue that humans have a basic right to food and that it should never be withheld. They differentiate feeding from medical treatment, regardless of the route of delivery. From their perspective, providing food and nutrition is our final communal link to the dying and demonstrates a respect for life. They believe that to continue to nourish and hydrate a hopelessly ill patient, even one who is permanently unconscious, is to preserve the "person." A further argument associates the painful sensations of hunger and thirst with physiologic status; those with this concern fear that withholding food and water will cause unbearable agony to the dying patient.

Others, however, argue that providing nutritional support to patients with a hopeless prognosis only prolongs the process of dying. Since any artificial means of nutritional support is intrusive and carries risks as well as benefits, they believe that it is properly viewed as a form of medical treatment; therefore the burdens and benefits of providing it should be assessed in each case, as is appropriate for all medical treatment. Their position is that a decision to forgo artificial means of nutrition and hydration is morally correct under circumstances in which providing it will not alter the irreversible downhill course of the underlying illness and will itself be disproportionately burdensome.

It is true that patients like Mrs. Franklin who are in a persistent vegetative state cannot experience the burden of any of the risks of continued feeding. However, neither can they realistically hope for benefits. The primary benefit conceivable for them is the recovery of consciousness and function, which has no reasonable possibility of occurring. A trial period of artificial feeding and hydration is obligatory when there is some hope of benefit to the patient. For this reason, the trials following Mrs. Franklin's first and second strokes were warranted, since the outcome for her was unclear. However, after two years, she is highly unlikely to recover or to improve function, and discontinuation of artificial nutrition and hydration may properly be considered in this second view.

Those who believe that respect for life requires that all available means be used to preserve it overlook that interventions that delay death do not necessarily connote respect for human life. Indeed, they may do just the opposite. At best, continued tube feedings will keep Mrs. Franklin alive until she succumbs to aspiration pneumonia, infection, or another stroke. Such efforts to delay death could violate the ethical precept, "Do no harm," especially where they increase physical discomfort or distress or negate the patient's wishes. Both medical and nursing codes of professional ethics specify a duty to respect human dignity. For example, the American Nurses' Association *Code for Nurses* states: "The nurse provides services with respect for human dignity and the uniqueness of the client. . . . Each client has the moral right to . . . accept, refuse, or terminate treatment."[1] In cases where treatment may prolong life but at great burden to the patient, the responsibility to respect human dignity and self-determination may be viewed as the primary obligation. Thus, the nurse's professional code of ethics could support withdrawal of nutrition and hydration in a case like that of Mrs. Franklin, especially where the previous value choices of the patient are known and where they indicate that the patient would want this.

A decision to limit or discontinue nutritional therapy can change the emphasis of health care from curing to caring. Those most intimately involved in providing care, the nursing staff, may differ from the family or physician in personal values, cultural and religious beliefs, background, and previous experiences. They may perceive non-feeding as not caring and as abandonment of the patient. For these reasons and also because they may have pertinent and important information about the patient and family, the nursing staff should be involved in the decisionmaking process. Further, nurses should always be involved in any decision with ethical implications that they are expected to implement. It is the duty of the health care team to communicate and work out any differences of opinion in a collaborative manner so that the patient's best interests can be protected and served. Disagreements should be recognized early and discussed. Persistent and thoughtful disagreements should be considered a warning to reconsider the decision.

When value differences will prevent a health care professional's continued involvement in care, the refusal should be made in advance, and an orderly transfer of care to another professional should be facilitated in a way that meets the patient's needs continuously. The refusal of Mrs. Franklin's nurse to participate is supported by the American Nurses' Association *Code of Ethics* which states: "If personally opposed to the delivery of care in a particular case, because of the nature of the health problem or the procedure to be used, the nurse is justified in refusing to participate. . . . The nurse withdraws from this type of situation only when assured that alternative sources of nursing care are available to the client" (p. 47).

The primary nurse believes that her personal integrity would be compromised if she were either to discontinue the tube feedings or provide supportive nursing care. However, honoring the request of the primary nurse not to be involved is difficult as a practical matter in this case because of the nursing home setting. Staffing patterns in most long-term care facilities, where only one professional nurse on each shift may be responsible for the care of all the patients in the facility, may preclude the orderly transfer of the nurse from this case. The "alternative sources of nursing care" may be unavailable, and Mrs. Franklin's nurse may be forced to choose between resigning or participating in care that violates her conscientious beliefs. The institution itself has a duty to its patients and its employees to provide a means for addressing and resolving such questions and to arrange for the orderly transfer of care from one provider to another.

In a nursing home, there is reasonable concern that a decision to discontinue food and water for one resident, if not understood in context, may unduly frighten other residents and may be misinterpreted by nonprofessional staff. Thus, when a facility cannot do this without risking the quality of care to the other residents, the institution is morally justified in declining to carry out the request and in giving the family the options of transferring the patient home or to another facility or of continuing treatment in the current facility. This may raise major difficulties that require legal resolution, however. The family might find that the need to adjust to a new setting and different health care providers during their mother's dying process would constitute a burden. Similarly, taking their mother home to die might be difficult for them. The family might have the option of hiring private nurses around the clock to care for their mother at the nursing home; however, the intense staff conflict over the decision to withdraw nutrition and hydration may make this solution untenable at this point.

There are actions that nursing homes and other health care institutions can take to help prevent the development of such difficult situations. During the hiring process, potential employees ought to be told about the kinds of care likely to be provided in the facility. Similar clarification is necessary for patients and families during the admission process. Staff education about policies that require collaboration of caregivers in ethical decisionmaking is essential. An ethics committee or consultation service to assist in decisionmaking should be made available. Finally, supportive services for staff and families are imperative.

The *Guidelines* recommend that artificial means of providing nutrition and hydration be viewed as medical interventions which may, under some circumstances, be forgone. [*See* Part Two: "Specific Treatment Modalities," Section C. "Medical procedures for supplying nutrition and hydration."] They suggest that when the patient lacks decisionmaking capacity, a surrogate should be identified to make treatment decisions for the patient. [*See* Part One: "Making Treatment Decisions," II., (3) "Identifying the key decisionmaker," (b) "Identifying a surrogate."] This surrogate should follow written advance directives or oral expressions of the patient's preferences or, if these are not available, should choose as would a reasonable person in the patient's circumstances, weighing burdens and benefits. [*See* Part One, II., (4) "Making the decision," (c) "The patient who lacks decisionmaking capacity."] The *Guidelines* note that the major consideration in deciding about treatment for those with irreversible loss of consciousness is whether a reasonable person in the patient's circumstances would find that the benefits to the patient as well as to the patient's family provided by treatment are outweighed by the burdens.

The *Guidelines* further recommend that institutions develop written policies regarding such decisions to forgo and provide nutrition and hydration. The *Guidelines* recognize the right of health care professionals to refuse to participate and their duty to provide for an orderly transfer of care. [*See* Part One, II., (8) "Objections and challenges," (e) "Withdrawal of health care professional or institution."] Referral to institutional ethics committees and, as a last resort, to the courts is recommended when ethical disagreements on the health care team cannot be resolved or the patient cannot be transferred to the care of another health care professional. Provision of support for members of the treatment team who provide care for dying patients is urged. Finally, the *Guidelines* specify that supportive care should be provided to the patient when life-sustaining treatment is withdrawn or forgone, thus preventing abandonment of the patient.

NOTE

1. American Nurses' Association (1978), "Code for nurses with interpretive statements (1976)." In *Perspectives on the Code for Nurses* (Kansas City, MO: ANA), p. 46.

13. Shadows from the Holocaust: The Case of Rachel and David

Rachel and David, a married couple who are survivors of a Nazi concentration camp, are seventy-eight and eighty. Their lives have focused on their experiences during the Holocaust, but in very different ways. Rachel has been embittered by it and has remained at home, never leaving it for any reason. For the past five years she has repeatedly expressed a desire to die; she does not feel that her marriage offers her a reason to live. David leads a fuller life and pursues many cultural activities outside their home. From time to time, he talks to community groups about his experiences in Nazi Germany. He, too, has been unhappy with his marriage.

Rachel has a history of rheumatic heart disease and depression. She was in relatively stable health until her most recent birthday, when she had an onset of atrial fibrillation and suffered an acute stroke. Following this, her neurologic condition deteriorated. She was only minimally responsive, moaned all day long, and made repetitive, purposeless movements. She did not speak, nor did she appear to understand when others spoke to her. She was unable to feed herself and required tube feedings to remain adequately hydrated.

David was profoundly upset by her acute deterioration and became totally devoted to her care. He visited Rachel every day and saw a hopeful sign in all of her movements. When doctors tried to explain to him that her prognosis was poor, he refused to accept this. After three months in the hospital, Rachel was placed in a nursing home.

Two days later, Rachel was returned to the hospital after she developed an aspiration pneumonia that required intravenous antibiotic therapy. It was necessary to restrain her during the course of her therapy because she pulled out her intravenous lines. She struggled endlessly to be removed from these restraints.

Rachel has remained in the hospital for six months, receiving intermittent courses of antibiotics for recurrent aspiration and urinary tract infections. Her neurologic condition has not improved, and she continues to resist the restraints. The house staff taking care of her has begun to feel that this woman is inadvertently being put through torture. Her terrible experience in the Holocaust has made them especially sensitive to her current situation. They suggest that no further antibiotic treatments be given to her. David, however, insists that Rachel would rather undergo the discomfort of the treatments than risk overwhelming infection and death. He accuses the staff of trying to kill Rachel, just like the Nazis.

If Rachel develops another infection, should it be treated with antibiotics or other antimicrobials? Why or why not?

Commentary by Bruce Jennings

The paradigmatic cases on forgoing life-sustaining treatment are those in which the patient, or the patient's surrogate, wishes to terminate treatment, while the health care providers or the health care facility resist the request and insist on continued treatment. In this case the roles are reversed: the physicians are saying enough is enough; the patient's husband is saying do everything to prolong life. The physicians are caught in a nasty bind. If they continue to treat Rachel's pneumonia aggressively, they will feel like torturers. If they don't, they'll seem, at least in David's eyes, like killers. Here the shadows from the Holocaust are long, and they come from both directions.

What we need desperately to hear is the voice of the patient. But Rachel's stroke has rendered her incapable of speaking for herself or taking part in the decisionmaking process. Apparently, and most unfortunately in this case, she has prepared no written advance directive to guide her care. Yet we do know that she has consistently expressed a desire to die during the past five years. One may reasonably ask, therefore, how meaningful and valuable prolonged life is for her and whether she would choose to undergo continued treatment if she could communicate her wishes. In struggling to remove her intravenous lines is she simply reacting to an irritating stimulus, or is she in fact communicating her wish to be allowed to die?

Finally, this case is exceptionally difficult because it involves the use of antibiotics rather than some more aggressive, invasive, and "extraordinary" or "heroic" form of life-sustaining treatment. It is interesting to note that the case focuses on the cessation of antibiotic therapy rather than the termination of artificial nutrition and hydration. These two treatment modalities are often set apart from other forms of life-sustaining interventions; some argue that it is never justifiable to withhold these treatments because to do so is patently to intend the death of the patient, and thus to cross the line between forgoing treatment (which may be acceptable) and euthanasia (which is not).

The first issue raised by the case, then, is whether or not antibiotic therapy is a mode of life-sustaining treatment that can ever be forgone. The second issue is on what basis one might justify forgoing treatment in Rachel's case. A third issue is whether David ought to serve as the surrogate in this case, and if so, whether or not his decision to continue treatment should be respected or overridden. A final question is whether ethical analysis can really make a difference in practice in a case like this. Readers of this case may want to consider whether in their own health care facility, it is likely that antibiotic therapy would actually be discontinued over the husband's objections, given the possibility of subsequent litigation, the anti-Semitic overtones this might create, and the media coverage such a lawsuit would be likely to generate.

The first two issues may be considered together. Generally speaking, an argument in favor of forgoing any form of life-sustaining treatment, including antibiotic therapy, requires a patient-centered justification. That is, it must be shown either that (*a*) the treatment in and of itself is unduly and disproportionately burdensome to the patient or that (*b*) the experience of the prolonged life that the treatment makes possible is unduly burdensome, given the patient's other underlying medical ailments and disabilities. Those who maintain that antibiotic therapy may never be forgone, unless it is virtually futile in curing a discrete life-threatening infection, tend to argue two points. First, they reject the notion that a justification for forgoing treatment may appeal to condition (*b*) above. That is, they reject the notion that the burdensomeness of life itself can provide a rationale for withholding or withdrawing a medically efficacious treatment. Second, in regard to antibiotic therapy in particular, they hold that it is never unduly burdensome in and of itself. This is an empirical claim about which medical experts disagree. It may be that repeated courses of antibiotics have debilitating and iatrogenic side-effects which produce appreciable suffering for the patient, even though they effectively stave off a particular life-threatening episode.

In this case, however, the main point of contention is not the burdensomeness or futility of antibiotic therapy *per se,* but the burdensomeness and quality of the experience of life that is prolonged by the therapy. To admit that antibiotics therapy is not in an ethically privileged class but may be ethically forgone under certain circumstances is to admit that, for some patients, death by pneumonia or some other massive infection is the death of choice. It is to be preferred over other forms of death that foreseeably await the patient down the road; and it is to be preferred over waiting for them.

How do these considerations apply to Rachel? This case is particularly difficult because Rachel is not "terminally ill" in any obvious sense of the term. Her death from pneumonia today will not spare her a slow, agonizing death from cancer tomorrow. Instead, her death from pneumonia today will spare her the continued indignity of physical restraints and the suffering created by her neurologically debilitated condition.

The problem in applying the patient-centered justification to this case is that we have to infer so much from Rachel's present behavioral patterns without being able to know exactly what state of consciousness or intentionality lies behind them. And we also have to infer a great deal from what we know about her past depression and her sense of the meaninglessness of her life. If David, her husband and life-long companion, were to agree that Rachel would not want to continue to live in her present condition, then we might feel more confident in making those inferences. But he does not.

What leads the house staff to arrive at their feeling that Rachel is "inadvertently being put through torture"? Is this an objective or "reasonable person" assessment of the pain and suffering associated with the antibiotic therapy and Rachel's physical restraints? Or is it perhaps a more esthetic response on their part, a reaction to the sheer horror and tragedy of the situation? Such a response would certainly be understandable. But is it an adequate basis upon which to decide that an otherwise viable patient should be allowed to die?

On the other hand, David's objectivity and his ability to apply the reasonable person standard in assessing Rachel's best interests do not exactly inspire confidence, either. Termination of treatment decisions are often a lightning rod where longstanding family tensions and feelings of guilt are discharged. When we expect surrogates objectively to evaluate the best interests of an incompetent patient, we are in fact asking them to perform a Herculean psychological and moral task. To achieve the objectivity of the reasonable person standard, the surrogate must be able to set aside his own personal values, beliefs, prejudices, hopes, and fears. He must adopt something like what the philosopher Thomas Nagel has called "the view from nowhere"; he must move in judgment and thought to a place detached from his own previous life history and the narrative of his relationship to the patient. If this, or something like this, were not our expectation, then we would have no way of making sense of the difference between those times when the surrogate is objectively assessing the patient's best interests and those times when the surrogate is projecting his own values and biases onto the patient. This difference is important because the moral legitimacy of the surrogate's decisionmaking authority hinges upon it.

This is a demanding ideal, to be sure. Indeed, it can't be more than an ideal, a theoretical limiting case that actual instances of surrogate decisionmaking approximate to a greater or lesser degree but can never fully attain. The "reasonable person" is a hypothetical construct, a fiction; she is no one and nowhere. But a surrogate decisionmaker, like David, is a concrete human being embedded in a thick web of social and historical relationship; he is someone somewhere. The question is how much latitude should the surrogate be allowed? How far short of the regulative ideal of objectivity must a surrogate fall before his decision should be challenged, reviewed by an outside body such as an institutional ethics committee or a court, and perhaps overruled? There is no doubt that David carries with him a very thick web of historical and personal meanings in his relationship to Rachel. But I do not see any clear-cut reason why his judgment as the surrogate in this case should be overridden. It is vitally important that a good relationship and good communications between David and the health care team be restored, for he must be prepared for other, and probably even more difficult treatment decisions that lie ahead. At the moment, though, the right course of action in this case is so ambiguous that we should err on the side of life. And David chooses life.

The *Guidelines* place antibiotic therapy on a moral par with other forms of life-sustaining treatment; they reject the notion that antibiotics can never justifiably be withheld. [*See* Part Two: "Specific Treatment Modalities," Section D. "Antibiotics and other life-sustaining medication."] In assessing the best interests of the patient in terms of the benefits and burdens of the therapy, the *Guidelines* also permit broad consideration of the patient's future life prospects and long-term suffering; they do not limit the question to the efficacy or futility of the treatment vis-à-vis a specific episode of infection. [*See* Part Two, Section D. "Antibiotics and other life-sustaining medication," II., (4) "Making the decision," (c) "The patient who lacks decisionmaking capacity," (3) "Or choose as a reasonable person in the patient's circumstances would."]

In this respect the *Guidelines* establish a framework within which a surrogate and the responsible health care professionals could ethically decide to forgo further antibiotic therapy. On the other hand, the *Guidelines* generally permit a fairly wide latitude of reasonable discretion for a surrogate, and they are based on a general presumption in favor of life-sustaining treatment when the patient's death is not imminent and unavoidable and when reasonable doubt exists concerning an incompetent patient's own treatment preferences. [*See* Preface.] In this case, since a disagreement exists between the attending physicians and the patient's surrogate, the *Guidelines* would authorize institutional review of the case and some attempt to mediate the dispute. But the *Guidelines* do not provide any clear-cut basis upon which David's judgment should be overruled, since Rachel did not leave any advance directives and since no other surrogate with an equally good knowledge of her values and wishes is present to contest David's decision.

Finally, the *Guidelines* would call upon the hospital in this case to permit any health care providers to withdraw from the case if they could not in good conscience continue to provide antibiotic therapy to Rachel, so long as adequate provision for her care was made. [*See* Part One: "Making Treatment Decisions," II., (1) "Underlying ethical values," (c) "The ethical integrity of health care professionals"; (8) "Objections and challenges," (e) "Withdrawal of health care professional or institution."]

14. The Old Man's Friend:
The Case of Carl Jurgen

Carl Jurgen is an eighty-three-year-old retired gold merchant who was admitted to a nursing home in March due to cognitive disabilities that prevent him from caring for himself. He had been a dashing figure throughout his life and had travelled widely across the world in the course of his business. He had never married and had no children. He had romanced several women whom he met during his travels and had maintained long-term relationships with two of them. His only living relative at this time is a niece who lives nearby.

Mr. Jurgen's laboratory tests on his admission to the nursing home were essentially normal. He was worked up for reversible dementia, but no treatable condition could be found. His cognitive function at that time was too limited to measure by standardized testing. Although he could say a few words clearly, they had no meaning. He was incontinent. Those caring for him felt that Mr. Jurgen adjusted to long-term care adequately.

In July, Mr. Jurgen began to eat a smaller amount of solid food. Nurses noted that his skin was fragile. Yet when he was examined, no new medical problem or abnormality could be found. Laboratory data showed that he had a marked anemia and that his serum albumin was reduced. These factors indicated that his overall condition and nutrition were not up to par. In addition, blood was found in his stools.

Soon after this, Mr. Jurgen developed a fever and had twitching of his limbs. He was sent to the hospital for treatment of "seizures." It turned out that he had a bladder infection that responded well to antibiotics. During this hospitalization, a liver scan, taken as part of a routine work-up, showed a large mass strongly suggestive of metastatic cancer. He was returned to the nursing home without further diagnostic tests.

The general picture of Mr. Jurgen at this time was of a frail, thin, and severely demented man who took pureed food listlessly and slept much of the time. He interrupted the quiet of the nursing home unexpectedly during day and night with episodes of screaming for which no cause could be found. The medical staff believed that there was a 90 percent probability that he had metastatic carcinoma of the colon. They felt that there was no realistic chance that his dementia was reversible.

His niece was saddened by his situation. She was concerned that his recent turn for the worse was caused by the disruptive effect of his hospitalization and asked that further hospitalization be avoided if possible. She wanted him kept comfortable.

It is now three weeks later. The day before yesterday, Mr. Jurgen would not eat dinner and was more sleepy than ever before. He seemed to be in no distress. His physician ordered serum electrolytes. They were returned yesterday and were normal, showing no dehydration, kidney failure, or severe glucose abnormality. Today, his food intake remains poor, and his temperature has risen to 102. This morning, his physician thought that he was breathing heavily and ordered a portable chest x-ray that was taken in bed for his comfort. It showed a small area of pneumonia.

Mr. Jurgen is likely to die in the next few days or weeks if his pneumonia is not treated. He is comfortable at present. Antibiotics might cure this infection or they might be fairly ineffective and just lengthen the process of dying. If he survives this episode of pneumonia, he will probably live for some months, have occasional pneumonias, and possibly develop severe anemia or bowel obstruction that will cause his death.

Mr. Jurgen's niece and the medical and nursing staff are discussing whether his pneumonia should be treated with antibiotics. If it is not, his niece wants to know what sort of care he would be given.

Do you think that Mr. Jurgen should be given antibiotic treatment for his pneumonia? Why or why not?

Commentary by Ellen Olson

Some might argue that antibiotics must at least be tried for patients in the face of a potentially life-threatening infection. Since antibiotics are readily available, inexpensive, and generally effective, many think that they must always be administered, even though there may be some other disease process that diminishes the degree of recovery that can be expected for a patient. In a situation where the patient has good venous access and an IV is easy to maintain, a trial of antibiotics to treat a pneumonia may not seem sufficiently burdensome to outweigh the experience of dying from increased secretions, hypoxia, and ultimately, respiratory failure. And when a patient responds very quickly, it may be difficult in retrospect to justify not having used antibiotics, despite the overall poor prognosis of the patient. It is when treatment fails or administration becomes difficult that we begin to question the presumption in favor of using antibiotics.

But there are situations where it is appropriate to consider even the simple administration of antibiotics a potential burden to the patient, despite its possible short-term efficacy. It is very likely that Mr. Jurgen would respond to antibiotic treatment, but to what end? What long-term goals would we be addressing in treating his acute infection? Is a death now from pneumonia preferable to one in a few months from a bowel obstruction or some other complication of his presumed metastatic carcinoma? Treatment in a lethargic patient who is not eating requires either a nasogastric tube or IV insertion. Both of these can be uncomfortable and have some attendant morbidity. The question of whether to use antibiotics, therefore, cannot be isolated from all other treatment questions and from a comprehensive view of Mr. Jurgen's situation.

The use of antibiotics should satisfy the basic premise that the possible benefits of treatment outweigh its relative burdens. When patients have the capacity to make a decision about this, the primary health care provider has an obligation to discuss treatment alternatives with them and to allow them the opportunity to accept or refuse treatment—unless there are public health issues at stake that mandate treatment. Although requests for clearly futile treatments need not be honored, the request of patients with capacity, but with an otherwise bleak prognosis, for treatment with only short-term efficacy should be honored. Such patient decisions should be nullified only on the basis of carefully worked out public and institutional policies that deal with questions of justice and equitable distribution of scarce resources. In patients without capacity, such as our patient, Mr. Jurgen, and in the absence of advance directives, medical decisions are usually made by surrogate decisionmakers in consultation with the primary health care provider and other members of the health care team. The choices that surrogate decisionmakers make should, in general, be more constrained than those of a patient deciding for himself, especially in the area of withholding therapies.

Patients who cannot speak for themselves must not only be protected against the indiscriminate practice of non-treatment but also against treatment that serves no useful purpose. Therefore, identifying the surrogate is one of the most important duties of the health care provider. The surrogate should be the person most familiar with the patient and with what he would have wanted if he could make his own choices. In this instance, the appropriate surrogate appears to be Mr. Jurgen's niece, although it might be reasonable to see if either of the two women with whom he had long-term relationships had any information regarding his preferences that might help the decisionmaking process. Family members are usually the people turned to for surrogate decisionmaking, but surrogates need not be restricted to family.

In the absence of advance directives, and presuming that Mr. Jurgen's niece has no specific information about what he would have wanted if he could participate in his care decisions, we must fall back on the "best interests" standard, that is, do what a "reasonable person" would want done in a similar situation based on a benefit versus burden analysis.

Age should not be a major consideration here. The same dilemma could occur in a forty-year-old woman with metastatic breast cancer. Dementia prevents Mr. Jurgen from deciding for himself and also makes it difficult to ascertain his level of suffering. The real significance of dementia lies in how it pertains to Mr. Jurgen's quality of life. Whenever possible, quality of life determinations should be made by the individual patient. What might seem a marginal or unacceptable quality of life to others might still be adequate to the patient and such that he or she would want it continued for as long as possible. There are situations, though, when the patient cannot decide for himself and the observer can reasonably assess the quality of a patient's life as below a minimally acceptable level for any human being. These instances include clearly irreversible and fatal conditions that are associated with extreme pain and suffering. We are in the process of working out a societal consensus about this that is grounded in respect for individuals and concern for their good, as it is essential to protect certain helpless groups of patients from burdensome and futile treatments. It is also essential to prevent misuse of the notion of quality of life that could lead to decisions based on the social worth of patients or their burden to society. [*See* Part Six: "Special Problems," IV. "Quality of Life."] This last point is also a reason why age and dementia *per se* should not serve as criteria for limiting treatment. [*See* Part Six: "Special Problems," V. "Age as a factor in decisionmaking."]

Once the surrogate is identified, the health care team must provide the information necessary to help the surrogate make a reasonable decision, relying as much as possible on what the surrogate thinks the patient would want done in this situation. We are assuming that Mr. Jurgen has a terminal process. A more definitive diagnosis would not change the picture enough to warrant the distress that could be created for Mr. Jurgen by hospitalization and the use of uncomfortable procedures to gather more information. At present, Mr. Jurgen is poorly responsive and, though breathing heavily, appears comfortable. His condition is not clearly causing suffering and is not clearly in its terminal stages. I believe that consideration of the benefits and burdens of treatment to Mr. Jurgen leads to a decision in favor of treatment.

Before this illness, Mr. Jurgen was responsive enough to take oral feedings to a degree that at least maintained hydration. He had episodes of crying out, but these did not seem to be related to physical suffering. Based on this information, I would argue that continued treatment would not be sufficiently burdensome to warrant withholding life-sustaining therapies. His most recent change in mental status, with increased lethargy and decreased food intake, may be secondary to his pneumonia and therefore reversible with antibiotic therapy. Further, the patient has not shown any clear-cut signs of bowel obstruction, and although his pneumonia may be a sign of that, it may also be an isolated incident, easily responsive to treatment. If any doubt exists in the mind of his surrogate about whether he would want to be treated, treatment would be the preferred option, for he may still have some positive life experiences. It should be emphasized, though, that a decision to treat at this time need not be irreversible. If the well-defined goal of returning Mr. Jurgen to his baseline of a few weeks ago is not reached quickly and without significant discomfort from IV's or nasogastric tubes, then the antibiotics can be discontinued once they become burdensome.

Not treating Mr. Jurgen with antibiotics could be interpreted as introducing another cause of death, especially if narcotics were required to make the patient in respiratory distress more comfortable. There are no guarantees that such an approach would not be construed as euthanasia. But if the intent is to minimize suffering and not to hasten death, the reasons are well-documented, and there is consent among surrogates and caregivers that this approach is consistent with the patient's wishes, not treating Mr. Jurgen would also be an acceptable decision. In the absence of clear directives from Mr. Jurgen that his current status is not satisfactory to him, however, I do not feel it is the preferred decision.

If this latter course were chosen on the basis of his clearly stated previous wishes, Mr. Jurgen should still get other comfort measures, including antipyretics, suctioning, oral hygiene (including moistening of the mouth and lips), turning and positioning, and sedation as needed. Oral feedings should be offered, on the premise that the patient might be experiencing hunger and thirst and would respond appropriately if that is so. Some might argue that food and water must be provided to the end of life for a multitude of moral and professional reasons. In Mr. Jurgen's case, this only could be done with nasogastric tubes or IV's. Artificial nutrition and hydration would only prolong the dying process, and there is no moral obligation to provide them. In fact, dehydration may be beneficial in a person with pneumonia, as it may decrease secretions and have some sedative effect. To hydrate Mr. Jurgen without providing antibiotics might make him more uncomfortable. The distinction must be made between addressing hunger and thirst by means of food and water which are comfort measures, and reversing physiological abnormalities by means of artificial nutrition and hydration.

The main strength of the *Guidelines* [*See* Part Two: "Specific Treatment Modalities," D. "Antibiotics and other life-sustaining treatment,"] in this case is that they not only help lay the groundwork for our discussion up to this point but they suggest a mechanism that would be helpful if agreement between surrogate and caregivers cannot be reached. That is an institutional ethics committee and a set of institutional guidelines that have been developed to deal cases like this. [*See* Part Five: "Policy Considerations," A. "Ethics Committees."] The committee could not only ensure that all relevant information is considered, but could also advise caregivers and surrogate and help them to settle any disputes before recourse to the courts seemed necessary. The *Guidelines* also suggest what would have been the preferred mechanism in this case, and that is the establishment of advance directives by Mr. Jurgen before he became incapable of making such difficult care decisions for himself. [*See* Part Three: "Prospective Planning" A. "Advance Directives."]

15. Gambling on Palliation:
The Case of Doris Van Cleve

"Hello. Sally? It's Dori.

"Just got back from the hospital. I saw the doctor and I ran all of those questions by him that we worked out. Yeah, it's really bad.

"The last time, he said that I have three choices. The first is to have extensive surgery. This time he called it 'a pelvic exenteration for uterine cervical cancer'. That means they'd take out part of my intestines, and then I'd have to wear one of those bags. That's called a 'colostomy'. I'd also have to have a hysterectomy. No more uterus. Then they'd take out my bladder. That would mean another bag so that my urine could be diverted externally. And finally they'd do a 'radical node dissection', which means that they'd take out all of the lymph nodes in the area of the uterus, along the aorta, and the vena cava. Yeah, Sally, heart stuff too. He said that all of this would give me a five per cent chance of a cure. That's right, five per cent.

"The second choice is surgery that's not as extensive. They'd still take out my uterus (I almost said, '*just* take out my uterus'!), but nothing else. Then they'd use radiation. No, Sally. He said I might have some side effects from the radiation, but usually there's no vomiting and all that misery. He confirmed that this is only what he called 'palliative'. It'll slow the cancer down, but it'll still kill me. I'd be more comfortable if I had this surgery until near the end and then things would get bad.

"The third choice is doing nothing. I'd die the earliest on this one. I'd bleed a lot and might get uremia—you know, my plumbing would stop working—and intestinal obstruction. He said that they'd do everything possible to keep me comfortable if I picked this third one, but it wasn't too pleasant. The problem is that the second choice—palliation—ends this way too. It just takes a little longer.

"When I told him at this visit that I had thought about it and that I was going with the second choice—palliation—he became very concerned. He said that he had strongly recommended the first choice and that he still does. He said that it's the only one that gives me a chance to live and that I ought to 'maximize my chances of survival'. Yeah, that's how he put it. I'm supposed to learn how to gamble now. And I've never even been to Las Vegas. The palliation stuff, he said, is a waste of time, as it'll get you anyway in the end. There's more to life than being made comfortable, he said. He told me that if it were his wife, he'd expect her to be a fighter, that I ought to try and beat this thing. He said that as a doctor, he is obliged to tell his patients that they ought to try to live, and he strongly believes that. That's what God put us on earth for.

"But I don't know. I'm not into gambling and prize fighting. I don't want to die, but I don't know if I want to live like that. I don't think that God expects me to have to go through all of that to stay alive.

"I told him that all of that surgery in the first choice doesn't seem worth it. But he said that it gives me a chance for life that none of the other choices do. And he said that my quality of life wouldn't be bad—that I'd be changing bags every day, but he's had patients who've been doing this for years, and they've learned to deal with it. Yeah. He said he'd put me in touch with a support group. I don't know if I could go through all of that for five per cent. No, he didn't say what the risks of the surgery itself were. I guess there goes my five per cent. No, don't worry about making it seem worse. I need to think through the whole thing carefully. The five per cent solution doesn't seem like a real solution.

"Listen. Could you come on over so that we can talk about it some more? Yeah, soon. Thanks."

Is palliation an ethically acceptable choice for Dori, since she has a chance to be cured? Should her physician have placed the responsibility for making a final decision in her hands?

Commentary by Ruth Oratz

This case raises several questions related to the role of palliative care in the management of terminal illness. In choosing which, if any, surgical procedure she wants, Doris is really choosing between competing values: on the one hand, the possibility (though low probability) of cure and prolongation of life, no matter what the burdens; on the other, a shorter life with perhaps less pain and suffering. This kind of choice is sometimes said to relate to a person's "quality of life." This neat, compact phrase implies that there is a single, objective definition of a good condition in which to live when, in fact, we have different ideas about what is meaningful and worthwhile in life. Each of us must rank our own values and preferences and weigh the relevant benefits and burdens offered to us and to others by each situation in order to determine what makes a life worth living.

Patients like Doris are faced with choosing between a variety of treatment plans, each of which carries different expectations for probability of cure and relief of pain and suffering, as well as different possibilities of complications and hardships. Is life always worth living no matter what the burdens—even if it would be a life that does not allow for participation in certain activities or realization of certain goals? Would living with a colostomy and ureterostomy impair Doris's ability to live a life that she would view as at least minimally good? Would it matter if she were a librarian or a ballet dancer? Could she learn to derive joy from new activities or to find meaning in different aspects of her life? Or are some kinds of life simply not acceptable, not worth living no matter what the benefits, such that any treatment that might sustain them could be forgone?

Some believe that it is wrong to weigh the burdens of life in a certain condition and that only the burden of the treatment itself should be considered in medical decisionmaking. They argue that it would be dangerous to define certain kinds of lives as not valuable for fear that this might encourage withholding treatment from large categories of patients on arbitrary grounds. Furthermore, they maintain that allowing quality of life issues to enter into treatment plans would sanction suicide, if not killing. One response to these objections is that quality of life issues are unavoidable. Even these objectors would concede that it is ethically appropriate to allow terminally ill patients to forgo treatment that might extend their lives because of the poor quality of life that such treatment would provide. Where is the fine line to be drawn between the burdens of treatment and the burdens of the condition that treatment produces? The issue becomes then, not whether to consider the quality of life, but what quality of life to consider too poor to justify maintaining by all available aggressive treatment. [See Part Six: "Special Problems," V. "Quality of Life."] This does not necessarily involve suicide or killing, for there is no desire that the patient die and no direct attempt to bring about death, but only a reluctant acceptance of the pathos of a situation that presents a tragic choice. [See Part Six: "Special Problems," I. "Terminating treatment, active voluntary euthanasia, and assisting suicide."]

In this case, Doris is offered the option of palliative surgery—perhaps a compromise between the extremes of accepting all treatment that offers even a remote chance of cure and refusing any treatment that would have even slightly unpleasant side effects. The goals of such palliative treatment include relief of pain and suffering, control of unpleasant symptoms, limiting the progression of disease, and affording maximum functional capacity. These are among the benefits to be considered by Doris in deciding whether to have palliative surgery.

What are the burdens of such care? By definition, palliative treatment does not aim to eradicate disease; cure cannot be anticipated. But there are often other concerns that patients like Doris have. If she chooses palliation rather than cure, will she lose the full support of her doctor? In "gambling away" her only chance for cure is she also gambling away treatment for the symptoms of her disease, help in coping with the physical, emotional, and financial complications of her illness? The answer to this question must emphatically be *NO*. In choosing palliative rather than curative treatment, the patient is not abandoning all hope of life, but is choosing one kind of life over another. She should be assured that she will not be deserted by her physician or any other member of the health care team as she leads that life. All health care providers have an obligation to continue to provide symptomatic relief of pain and suffering, emotional reassurance, physical contact, and social support to the patient who chooses palliative, rather than curative therapy. [*See* Part Two: "Specific Treatment Modalities," E. "Palliative care and the relief of pain," I. "Introduction."]

Are there other burdens associated with palliative treatment? Sometimes palliative surgery may itself be risky or disfiguring, sometimes it may only delay the appearance of painful or distressing symptoms that would then require more surgery or more intensive medical therapy, or sometimes it may result in new, unforeseen complications. Palliative medical treatment includes the administration of drugs which themselves may have side effects. For example, at times chemotherapy (or radiation therapy) might be given to control the pain and discomfort of cancer—without intent to cure. However, these drugs could cause nausea, vomiting, hair loss, and other unpleasant side effects. Patients must choose between the side effects of such palliative treatment and the symptoms of their disease—shortness of breath, pain, bleeding, paralysis.

In other circumstances, narcotics may be required for pain relief. These drugs also have side effects. Some health care providers and patients believe that narcotic use for analgesia leads to addiction. They perceive this as an undesirable burden and consequently withhold narcotics. In fact, patients do not become "addicts" when given doses adequate to relieve and prevent pain. Distressing symptoms of withdrawal are experienced when narcotics are abruptly discontinued, but this should never occur in patients who require medical treatment for painful conditions. If anything, we force patients to demand more drugs when they are undertreated, rather than overtreated!

An important side effect of narcotics is lethargy and/or somnolence. Patients will sometimes have to choose between complete pain relief and toleration of some pain in order to remain awake and alert. Narcotics and other analgesics may also sometimes suppress respiration. In a patient with respiratory insufficiency, this may be perceived as hastening death when this is not the intention. Once again, patients, surrogates, and the health care team must consider all of the benefits and burdens of a given treatment in deciding how to apply it. It would not be unethical to administer doses of narcotics that suppress respiration while relieving pain if the patient (or surrogate deciding on behalf of the patient) considers the benefits of pain relief to outweigh the burdens of potential respiratory suppression and/or arrest.

When is it appropriate to consider palliative treatment plans? Palliative care should be considered for all patients who choose to forgo the use of life-sustaining treatment. Patients known to be dying or terminally ill and those suffering from acute or chronic illnesses from which there is no longer a chance of recovery who decide against aggressive treatment should certainly be offered all modalities that might effectively treat their symptoms, relieve pain, and, if possible, restore functional capacity. Other patients who may be seriously ill or significantly impaired, but who have some chance of cure, may also decide to forgo life-sustaining treatment. These patients, like Doris, should be offered palliative treatment as an alternative. It must, however, be recognized that some patients may opt to forgo even palliative care. This choice should be subject to the same *Guidelines* used for forgoing life-sustaining treatments.

A final point raised by this case is the importance of planning—planning in advance. It is likely that no matter which option Doris chooses, she will ultimately face further complications and new symptoms related to the growth and spread of her cancer. She and her physician will be best prepared to deal with these and to choose from among future therapeutic and palliative options if they plan ahead now, while Doris is still relatively well and able to decide for herself. [*See* Part Two: "Specific Treatment Modalities," Section E. "Palliative care and the relief of pain," II., (9) "Special comments," (b) "Developing a plan for palliative care and pain relief."] Medical decisionmaking is a team effort guided by the patient. The patient, her family and close friends, her doctors and nurses as well as other members of the health care team must work together to develop the most appropriate plan for that patient.

16. Morpheus or Death:
The Case of Nicholas Miklovich

Nicholas Miklovich is a fifty-two-year-old man with a widespread squamous cell carcinoma of the lung. He lives alone at home. He has a forty pack-year history of smoking and chronic bronchitis. His bone pain has become severe in the past few weeks. Although he is now taking 120 mg. of morphine orally every three to four hours, he remains quite uncomfortable.

If any of the following considerations applied, how would they affect a decision about Mr. Miklovich's morphine dose?
1. A trial dose of 180 mg. of morphine is effective in relieving pain but precipitates wheezing and labored breathing. Regular use of that dose might bring about respiratory insufficiency and even death. Trials with alternative narcotics run into the same problem.
2. Mr. Miklovich is found by a neighbor, confused and in pain and is taken by ambulance to a hospital. The physician who treats him there is concerned that the patient is on his way to addiction.
3. Hospice admission is available and undertaken. It is found that the only way to keep Mr. Miklovich comfortable is by having him sedated to the point of unconsciousness until he dies.

Commentary by Joanne Lynn

All of the possible courses suggested in this case raise the problems of balancing undesirable side effects with the pursuit of comfort for a person who is near death. Mr. Miklovich's situation is one marked by a very short prognosis, irrespective of treatment. While the medical facts presented are not extensive, "widespread" squamous cell carcinoma of the lung implies that he is likely to have severe weakness, bone pain, metastases to at least a few vital organs, and a lifespan of no more than a few months, possibly no more than a few weeks. His medical situation is complicated by the chronic obstructive lung disease, and his social situation is complicated by living alone.

1. *Respiratory complications from pain control*. If the first of the listed considerations applied, he would be having a bronchospastic (or asthmatic) response to morphine. This is uncommon, and it is even more uncommon that it cannot be avoided with substitute narcotics. However, when it occurs, it poses a serious dilemma: the treatment of choice for the most troubling symptom causes a side effect that is even more troubling to the patient than the original symptom. Neither being in pain nor feeling as though he is being suffocated is likely to be an acceptable endpoint for Mr. Miklovich. Possible alternatives at this point would include trying "second-line" treatments for the pain, such as radiation, nerve blocks, and non-narcotic analgesics, or trying to suppress the patient's asthmatic response with inhalant treatments, steroids, and bronchodilator drugs. Only if none of these is appropriate or effective would the physician and patient be left with a real dilemma.

As a practical matter, the short time course of the patient's illness and the likely changes in his mentation and physical condition in the days or weeks necessary to evaluate the above possibilities are likely to foreclose the possibililty of ever having to confront the dilemma in its full force. More likely, a day-to-day balance will be struck as each of the possibilities is tried in the context of still trying to keep all symptoms to a minimum and trying to adjust remedies to the changing situation of the patient.

One serious aspect of this situation is likely to be consideration of the patient's location for treatment. Virtually all of the potential treatments could be done at home or in an out-patient setting if the patient had a great deal of support from family and friends and especially if he had a capable live-in primary caregiver. However, they will be difficult and sometimes risky if the patient is trying to manage alone. In fact, the simple trajectory of his disease will make it difficult to manage at home alone for much longer, even if he were not having difficulties with pain management. If he is hospitalized, it is fairly likely that he would be too weak to manage back at home by the time a stable care plan was devised. If he has no other option to being at home or in hospital, he will have to be aware of the significance of the choice.

Certainly, any existing advance directives need updating at this juncture. This patient is now at high risk of becoming incompetent in the next few weeks, or even the next few days. If there is any doubt about his preferences with regard to treatment or if there are tasks yet to be done in preparation for his death, this would certainly be the time for Mr. Miklovich to attend to them. Especially in the setting of a person living alone, he needs to name an appropriate surrogate, if that is possible, and that surrogate needs to be made aware of the situation.

If, just to accept the "hardest" case, the only effective treatment for Mr. Miklovich's pain carries with it the likelihood of an earlier death due to side effects it seems that common sense and the *Guidelines* would dictate that the issue should be understood as choosing the least undesirable of two treatments with undesirable features. If the patient has a clear preference for full relief of pain despite the risk of precipitating respiratory insufficiency, that option should be made available. [*See* Part Two: "Specific Treatment Modalities," Section E. "Palliative care and the relief of pain," I. Introduction."] If it is possible, and if the patient prefers it, these options should be made available at home, though I would estimate that home care in this situation would rarely be possible given current health care structuring and insuring policies.

2. *Mental complications from pain control.* If, instead, Mr. Miklovich became confused while at home and then an Emergency Room physician became concerned about addiction, the following considerations would apply. First, the source of the confusion needs to be evaluated. Confusion is ordinarily troubling to the patient and removes the patient from a controlling role in health care, so it is almost always best for acute confusion to be examined quickly and carefully. In this situation, the patient may have easily reversible causes for confusion and is already in a setting where these can readily be evaluated. If confusion arises from inadequate oxygenation, dehydration, high calcium, or some other source that can be remedied fairly simply and if no objection by the patient is known in advance (which creates an obligation for the E.R. physician to contact the primary care physician in order to ascertain this), then these potential sources should be quickly evaluated and those that are identified should promptly be treated. If this restores Mr. Miklovich to his usual state of mental health, then he will be back in control of future decisions, able to reconsider the appropriateness of continued treatment (or repeated treatment if the problem should arise again), and able to decide the issue of whether to give up living alone.

If treatment does not restore adequate mental clarity or if evaluation discovers causes that are not treatable, then one hopes that adequate advance directives are available. Certainly, it will be of great help if the primary physician has already been in touch with an appropriate surrogate or if the outlines of appropriate care from this time until death have been clarified with the patient prior to this event. [*See* Part Three: "Prospective Planning," I. "Introduction."] If advance plans suffice, there will be no crisis in the decisionmaking. If there have been no advance plans and there is no one appropriate to be the patient's surrogate, the kind of supplemental procedure recommended in the *Guidelines* will have to be used. [*See* Part One: "Making Treatment Decisions," II., (3) "Identifying the key decisionmaker," (c) "The patient who lacks a ready surrogate."] In some states, the procedure required may actually extend to presenting Mr. Miklovich's situation to a court and asking a judge to name a stranger to make his decisions for him. Perhaps a judge may also have to be involved before an order against resuscitation can be written. Even if state law is not so onerous, the *Guidelines* suggest that the hospital have in place a procedure that ensures that the patient has a personal advocate overseeing the decisions made in order to ensure that they are in line with the patient's preferences and with his best interests.

If the physician is working in an institution that has not taken on this responsibility, the physician will have to seek to ensure that this patient whose own views are not known will have good decisions made and good decisionmaking practices utilized. While this might mean electively taking the matter to court, it is at least possible that the physician could construct adequate safeguards for the patient's civil rights by making efforts to involve family and friends, by obtaining consultations, and by convening an *ad hoc* ethics committee of knowledgeable caregivers, concerned friends and family, and persons with specific skills in ethics, law, or the patient's religion.

As a footnote to the real issues above, it should be clear that the physician's fears of addiction are absolutely irrelevant and misleading. The patient will certainly be physically dependent upon narcotics in the sense that sudden withdrawal could lead to unpleasant (but not dangerous) side effects. Gradual withdrawal would lead to no side effects. But withdrawal at all is unlikely to be appropriate, and provision of the narcotics in medical contexts does not cause antisocial, criminal, or self-destructive behaviors.

3. *Unconsciousness as a side effect of pain relief.* If the only troubling issue that arises during Mr. Miklovich's care is that of having to accept unconsciousness in order to avoid severe pain, this is a morally acceptable course. [*See* Part Two: "Specific Treatment Modalities," Section E. "Palliative care and the relief of pain," I. "Introduction."] The trade-off, of course, must be discussed in advance with Mr. Miklovich, and it must be clear that no less severe mental disability is possible. Then, sedation to achieve pain relief is good medicine and raises no particular moral concerns. It may be that a brief life of nearly continuous sedation is not of great merit, even though it is better than any other life that can be made available. And some patients might prefer deliberate overdosage so as to bring death earlier. However, continuous sedation achieves a humane and compassionate period of dying for patient, caregivers, and family without precipitating the very serious concerns about "slippery slopes" that arise with acceptance of direct killing. Therefore, sedation is the best policy in the unusual instance of pain so severe that it cannot be relieved while still keeping the patient awake.

Part Three

Prospective Planning: Advance Directives

17. Poetic License:
The Case of Theo

Theodore Lownik Library
Illinois Benedictine College
Lisle, Illinois 60532

Theodore was a seventy-three-year-old former high school teacher who had always been in excellent health. He continued to lead an active life after retiring eight years ago. He performed in plays in his retirement community and loved to have friends over for musical "jams" in which he played his banjo. Theo's teaching speciality had been English literature, and he was pleased to have the time to do his own writing now.

Although he had never been seriously ill, Theo was concerned about the prospect of prolonged illness that would require him to "live on machines." He had talked about this with his two brothers, his sister, friends, and physician, and had signed both a durable power of attorney and a "Living Will." The former designated his sister as his surrogate should he become unable to make medical care decisions. The "Living Will" indicated that he did not want to receive heroic treatment should he become terminally ill. The "Living Will" form seemed sterile to him, so he attached a rather whimsical sonnet to it that he had written. It read:

> I've been told by those more wise than I
> That man alone among the life of earth
> Has knowledge that one day he'll surely die
> By laws of nature writ before his birth.
> No hope to change such laws do I maintain,
> But only that my final passing on
> Be unencumbered by much fruitless pain,
> By tubes that do not suit a former don.
> Please do no deeds that cannot stop the flow
> Of life to death. But when my time is here
> Omit all tests and codes that say "Go slow,"
> Intensive care with costs that are too dear.
> Let me depart without machines and knife
> That only will prolong a hopeless life.

Everyone was surprised when Theo suffered what was probably a myocardial infarction (a heart attack) and had to be taken to an Emergency Room. Tests determined that he had suffered third degree heart block, and he was admitted to the Cardiac Care Unit of the hospital. Theo gave permission for additional tests, but when his physician wanted to put in a pacemaker, he refused and told him he didn't want "all those machines." The physician responded, "Oh, it isn't such a big deal to put in a pacemaker; it's when they start intubating you that you have something to worry about." Theodore hesitantly agreed to the procedure. However, shortly after it, his blood pressure dropped precipitously, he became severely short of breath, and he was intubated.

That evening Theo pulled out his tube; he was re-intubated. During the next few days, he became progressively weaker, confused, and disoriented. He no longer knew where he was, and sometimes did not recognize his visitors. His physician wanted to do a cardiac catheterization. Theo, however, refused permission. The physician believed that Theo was without decisionmaking capacity at this point, and so asked his sister for permission to do the catheterization. Theo's sister produced the "Living Will" that he had signed three months earlier, as well as his poem and durable power of attorney. She told the physician that Theo had made it clear that he did not want "all of these measures."

The physician said that "Living Wills" represent decisions made by people in healthy situations, and that they should not be recognized in a medical situation that a patient has never previously experienced. They are also too vague, he told her, to be of much help in determining what treatments a patient would want. He believed that it would be a mistake not to give Theo aggressive treatment now, for his prognosis was not hopeless. He was not at the point of "final passing on" about which he had written in his sonnet.

Theo's brothers, who were also present during the discussion with Theo's physician, told him that he should do whatever was necessary to save Theo's life. His sister, however, insisted that Theo's wishes should be respected and that he should only be given comfort measures.

Should the physician accede to Theo's sister and provide him with supportive care only?

Commentary by Cynthia B. Cohen

As they have seen the lives of critically ill relatives and friends maintained by remarkable new medical techniques, in some instances beyond a point that they would want for themselves, and in others not long enough, individuals have been writing "Living Wills." In these and other treatment directives, they have indicated to future health caregivers the kind and degree of treatment that they would want should they enter certain medical conditions and be unable to express their values and preferences. "Living Wills" are most frequently used to direct the cessation of life-sustaining treatment when people are terminally ill and near death. However, they need not be restricted to such situations. They can also be used to ensure that aggressive treatment is ended in a broader range of circumstances or that the treatment is provided in stated circumstances. Durable powers of attorney are becoming increasingly important as an additional kind of advance directive, generically known as a proxy directive, in which individuals appoint a surrogate to make treatment decisions for them should they become unable to decide for themselves.

The basic premise behind the use of these advance directives for medical treatment is that people have certain reflective values, beliefs, and preferences about the way in which they want to live and die that should be honored, even when they cannot speak for themselves. Approval of the use of these directives in our society reflects the high respect that we have for individual choice and self-determination, as well as for the communal values that individuals tend to adopt and make their own. We recognize the concern of physicians about the validity and appropriateness of treatment decisions made by patients in the abstract and acknowledge that people might want to choose in a different way from that which they had imagined once they are in a concrete situation. However, we also realize that if people no longer have the capacity to choose at that time, the best that we can do for them is to respect the kinds of choices that they made when they could decide.

Even though Theo had been leading a full, creative, and active life, he had the wisdom to realize that his circumstances could change. Therefore, he made certain decisions about the use of life-sustaining treatment in case he should be unable to indicate his preferences about this. Theo was no slouch. Not only did he make out a durable power of attorney, but a "Living Will" accompanied by an explanatory sonnet. Since we are not told of special terms that he wrote into his "Living Will," it is reasonable to assume that it follows the lines of most and that he does not wish to receive life-sustaining procedures should he become terminally ill and near death. An analysis of Theo's sonnet confirms this, for it refers to knowledge that "he'll surely die," his "final passing on," "the flow / Of life to death," and "a hopeless life." While this may not wholly overcome his physician's concern about the vagueness of treatment directives, it clearly indicates Theo's thoughts about the degree of treatment that he wishes to receive when he is irrevocably dying.

Theo, however, is not irrevocably dying. There is no reason to consider whether life-sustaining treatment should be withdrawn from him at this point. Further, Theo is not in any condition that is cousin to terminal illness for which reasonable people have been known to refuse treatment in advance. He is not in a persistent vegetative state, or suffering from extremely severe and irremediable mental and/or physical disability accompanied by acute pain. The question whether life-sustaining treatment should be ended for Theo, therefore, is irrelevant at this time.

That Theo made his sister his surrogate in his durable power of attorney does not mean that she can make any treatment decision for him that she wishes if he is incapacitated. The parameters of her decisions on his behalf are limited by his previous wishes or, if these are not known, by what would be viewed as in his interests at this time by reasonable persons. After all, it is Theo's right to privacy that his sister would be exercising if he has lost the capacity to make treatment decisions, not a right of her own to make decisions for him. In light of his treatment directives, it is premature for her to consider the withdrawal of life-sustaining treatment. She seems to have misunderstood either her brother's prognosis or else the treatment preferences that he expressed in his "Living Will" and sonnet.

If Theo's sister persists in wanting life-sustaining treatment withdrawn after she is again told that his condition is not terminal, her decision should be challenged. Some institutional mechanism should be available through which Theo's caregivers and brothers can seek review of her choice. This would help to protect Theo's well-being and autonomy, and could bring about a resolution of the matter before it became necessary to resort to the courts. An institutional ethics committee would provide a mediating force that could foster a decision in accord with Theo's previously expressed wishes. Such a group could help avoid placing Theo's sister and his physician and brothers in an adversarial relationship that would be damaging to Theo's future care. The institution has a responsibility to see to it that some such body is available for consultation and review in cases like Theo's. [*See* Part Five: "Policy Considerations," Section A. "Ethics committees."]

The uncertainty in this situation is not created exclusively by the vagueness of patient directives, as Theo's physician believes. There are numerous other uncertainties involved, including whether the medical prognosis is accurate. The determination of whether a critically ill patient is irreversibly ill and near death is notoriously difficult. Some physicians are reluctant to forgo the chance of a one-in-a-million miracle for their patients and, consequently, tend to disregard the likelihood that their patients are dying. The possibility of medical misjudgment should be considered by an institutional body not only when it can result in the unneccessary death of a patient, but also when it can result in the unnecessary prolongation of the dying process of a patient. While it is preferable to err on the side of life, it is better not to err in the first place.

If we assume that Theo's physician is correct and that his condition is not hopeless, the treatment decision that must be made right now is whether he should be catheterized. Theo's ability to make this decision appears seriously diminished, for he is "confused and disoriented" and is only intermittently aware of where he is and who others are. However, Theo's physician has an obligation not to assume that Theo cannot decide without carefully considering whether this is so. If, after testing and consultation with others who are experts in the evaluation of patient decisionmaking capacity, and after meeting any other requirements set by the institution, it is determined that Theo does not have the capacity to make a decision about catheterization, then it is appropriate to have Theo's sister decide. (Of course, this must be subject to a *caveat,* for, if Theo's physician is correct, his sister has already made one serious error in judgment.) If it is determined that Theo has the capacity to make this decision, consideration should be given to whether he is laboring under a misconception. He may mistakenly think that he is near death because of the off-hand comment of his physician about the seriousness of intubation. If this is the case, the physician should attempt to reverse this error. If, after this, Theo continues to assert that he does not want to be catheterized, he should not be catheterized.

The *Guidelines* recommend that responsible health care professionals should view advance directives as an expression of the considered wishes of their patients and should respect them. [*See* Part Three: "Prospective Planning," Section A. "Advance Directives."] Such written directives have been endorsed by statute in many states. Not only written, but oral directives have been given common law recognition in the courts of several states as well. The courts have generally been willing, indeed, eager to allow wishes expressed by patients when they had the capacity to make treatment decisions govern their care. Ethically, respect for the reflective value choices of persons requires that the preferences of patients with capacity be followed unless these would lead to serious injustice to other patients or would violate certain other values that are at the heart of a community based on such respect.

The conscientious physician who wishes to follow the wishes of patients may find it difficult to interpret a treatment directive after a patient has lost capacity. Treatment directives must be both general and flexible, so that they can cover classes of circumstances about which the patient is concerned and yet meet changes in the patient's condition. This sometimes leads to confusion about when a patient means the directive to become effective and what conditions and kinds of treatment it covers. It is important for caregivers to consult with surrogates who know the now-incapacitated patient well to ascertain whether the patient meant the treatment directive to apply in the current situation. If the patient has not developed a proxy directive and there is no court-appointed surrogate, the *Guidelines* recommend that the primary physician "find the person who is most involved with the patient and most knowledgeable about the patient's present and past feelings and preferences" to interpret the patient's wishes. [*See* Part One: "Making Treatment Decisions," II., (3) "Identifying the key decisionmaker," (b) "Identifying a surrogate."] Together, they can develop a treatment plan for the patient that respects his or her basic values and beliefs and that is directed toward the patient's welfare.

18. "Macho Man":
The Case of Antonio Ruiz

"I told him that he had stomach cancer and that it had spread. I felt really bad having to tell him so close to Christmas, but he needed surgery, and it couldn't wait until after the holidays. He was only twenty-eight years old. He took it very well, though maybe he didn't realize just how bad it was. He said, 'I'm in great shape. I work out at the gym and kick the ball around in the neighborhood. They call me "Macho Man." Just get it out of there, and I'll be O.K.'

"Antonio came from a large, close family. They were always with him. I knew that I was in for trouble when I had to tell them. They were waiting outside the door, and I wished I were in Singapore—wherever that is. When I told them, they were really upset, and they were getting him upset, too, so the nurse and I finally got them to leave.

"The next day, the surgeons did a resection with a thoracic esophago-gastric anastomosis.[1] Then he had three months of chemo and radiation. He did pretty well, except for the complication of some intermittent esophageal stricture.[2]

"Six months later, Tony came back while I was rotating through the service again. He looked paler and thinner and complained of "stomach troubles." But he said he was still out there tossing the ball around with the guys in the neighborhood. His alkaline phosphatase was elevated, but the CT scan was inconclusive.[3]

"In September he came in with vomiting and was found to have gastric outlet obstruction.[4] A thoraco-abdominal exploration confirmed extensive recurrence in the pericardium, stomach, and thoraco-abdominal midline structures.[5] They did a bypass gastro-jejunostomy, and put a jejunal feeding tube in.[6] Tony took all this pretty well, although he looked terrible. I kept remembering that they used to call him 'Macho Man' in the neighborhood. They gave him an appropriate name.

"Things got worse. He was having a lot of chest pain, so we started him on narcotics. At the beginning of October, we placed a Hickman catheter[7] for chemo. He had persistent tachycardia, and his liver function tests were off the wall, so we started a five-day course of cis-platinum-5FU.[8] He continued to deteriorate. He developed a fever with progressive pulmonary infiltrates[9]; we treated it with antibiotics.

"Tony began to get depressed. Part of me was surprised. The other part wasn't. He couldn't be 'Macho Man' forever. Then Tony sprang it on me. He said he wanted to be one of those 'No Codes', that he didn't want us pumping on his chest and breaking some ribs to keep him alive. He just wanted to go if he stopped breathing. His mother was there, and she wanted to know what this 'No Code' was, so I told her. I talked to my attending about what Tony said. She told me to give him more of a chance to respond to the chemo and antibiotics. I suggested that we talk to Tony now so that when he went, it'd be the way he wanted. She told me that he was depressed and that I should learn to keep more distance from my patients.

"Then he arrested. It was probably from the narcotics and aspirating vomit. He had this grey-green pasty look. We ran a code. I thought he'd die right then. Maybe I even thought that he should. But he didn't. We put in an endotracheal tube to help him breathe and sent him to the ICU. His pulmonary function deteriorated in the next few days. Chest X-rays showed chemical pneumonitis and pneumonia. Tony couldn't be weaned from the respirator and needed continuous narcotics. He was getting wild and was bucking the ventilator; the drugs helped knock him out.

"By the fifth day in the ICU, we all agreed that he had had it. Mrs. Ruiz must have overheard us talking—or maybe she just guessed—but she came over to me and said that it was time to stop the machine. She knew from what he said to me a few weeks before that he wouldn't want to go on this way. My attending said she'd talk to the ICU administrator and to the Chief of Staff about it.

"It was then that we found out that there was a problem because Tony had what they called 'decisionmaking capacity'. Would you believe it? According to hospital policy, if he wasn't able to decide, we could stop support, provided that his surrogate or closest relative asked. But since he 'had capacity', we would have to stop the drugs, wake him up, and ask him whether he wanted to be allowed to die with or without a machine. That would be crazy. Why make him miserable by waking him only to ask him how he wanted to die?

"We talked to his mother and father. They didn't want to have the drugs stopped. We went along with them, but it meant we couldn't take him off the respirator. Tony died right before Christmas. He was still attached to the machine."

Why did this outcome result? Was there anything that the resident, staff, or hospital administration could have done to avoid it? Should they have?

NOTES

1. an operation in which most of the stomach is removed and the esophagus is attached to the remainder of the stomach

2. a narrowing of the esophagus that makes it difficult to swallow food
3. the cancer has spread to the bone
4. a blockage where the stomach joins the small intestine
5. spreading into the chest and abdomen
6. an operation to bypass the obstruction; a feeding tube was inserted into the small intestine on the other side of the obstruction
7. a permanent intravenous line for the administration of chemotherapeutic agents
8. a chemotherapeutic agent
9. X-ray shows non-lung tissue in the lung

Commentary by Michael C. Cantor

This common case scenario is an excellent illustration of an unfortunate outcome when patients with illnesses that place them at serious risk are not given the opportunity to discuss treatment goals and options with their caregivers when they have the capacity to make decisions. All too often, it is only when a crisis intrudes and it is too late to consult with patients that life-and-death choices must be made. Physicians, who are trained to provide all available aggressive treatment for their patients, find it difficult to carry on frank conversations with critically ill patients about the range of treatment alternatives available—including those that are not curative. It seems contrary to their way of functioning professionally to accept that, in some situations, it is right not to provide aggressive measures and to allow patients to die. Some may project their own fears and moral values onto patients and rationalize this by saying that patients cannot understand the complexities of the illness or would be harmed by open discussion. As a consequence, they may veer away from broaching options that involve withdrawing or withholding aggressive treatment and find themselves in a difficult ethical, medical, and legal dilemma of a sort that is posed by Tony's case.

No one talked to Tony about his various treatment options and goals fairly early in his illness, although they knew that his long-range outlook was poor. Perhaps the resident identified with Tony as the attending physician claimed, since they were similar in age, and this made discussion of his cancer even more difficult than is ordinarily the case. That the resident wanted to avoid the discussion is reflected in his statement, "I knew I was in for trouble" and in his admission that he wished he were far away. Perhaps the lack of open discussion of Tony's outlook early in treatment was correct because it would have been counterproductive so soon after diagnosis. Tony, with his strong denial, might not have tolerated talking about an illness that impinged on his masculinity. Indeed, some would argue that it might have been positively detrimental to him and might have shortened the year-long extension of life that he eventually had. Yet it is not often the case that patients are harmed by careful consideration of their alternatives. Most can talk about important aspects of their illness and want to do so. Although the approach to each patient will vary, patients should be given the opportunity to discuss their future treatment options and preferences and to designate surrogates at a point in their illness when they indicate that they are ready to do so.

It became obvious during the course of his treatment that Tony had reached such a point when he raised the issue of being coded. It was inappropriate for the attending physician to dismiss his statement about this and to ignore the resident's suggestion that they plan for Tony's dying. It is difficult for residents to challenge decisions of attendings with which they disagree, for they (realistically) feel that their professional future may be put in jeopardy. However, it is possible for them to develop a support group of other residents, nurses, and caregivers of like mind who can pursue the matter with attendings through reasonable persuasion for the sake of the patient. In some institutions, ethics committees provide a non-threatening forum in which to discuss and resolve differences of opinion about when and what patients should be told by their caregivers. [*See* Part Five: "Policy Considerations," Section A. "Ethics Committees."]

The real problem in Tony's case was not that a deliberate decision was not made to discuss his condition and options with him, but that no explicit decision either way seems to have been made at all. It was simply assumed that there should be no discussion of the possibility that Tony might want to forgo certain life-sustaining treatments at some point. When Tony eventually broke through this taboo and volunteered his preference not to be resuscitated should he arrest, this was rejected as the product of depression. Some physicians who have difficulty in accepting the irrevocability of a life-threatening illness may feel that patients who do accept this must be suffering from emotional problems that impair their decisions. However, patients are presumed to have the capacity to make decisions unless there is clear evidence to the contrary. Depression alone does not render them incapable of making treatment choices. It should not have been assumed without further evaluation that Tony's emotional reaction meant that he could not choose whether he wanted to receive life-sustaining treatment.

A decision about whether to discontinue ventilator support had to be made for Tony at a time when his capacity to make a decision was in question. This precipitated a conflict between the value of patient autonomy, which hospital policy said could only be achieved by awakening Tony and exposing him to great suffering, and the value of beneficence, which his parents could only view under these circumstances as requiring that he be kept sedated and maintained on the ventilator. In my opinion, given the hospital policy, attempts should first have been made to withdraw some of the medication from Tony without allowing his decisionmaking capacity to be compromised by extreme pain and suffering so that he could consider whether he wanted to have ventilator support withdrawn. If this was not possible, it would have been reasonable to conclude, contrary to hospital policy, that Tony did not have the capacity to decide and that a surrogate had to make a decision for him. Tony would have lacked capacity either because medication could not be withdrawn from him without severe pain and suffering or because of that very pain and suffering. The hospital policy seems flawed in that it did not consider these possibilities.

While it is important for hospitals to have a policy in place about stopping the use of ventilators, the institutional administrators in this case interpreted their hospital's policy very narrowly, so that respirators would rarely be withdrawn. The policy apparently stipulated that patients whose underlying mental capacities were presumably still intact had to be considered capable of making treatment decisions if they were sedated. It also required that when a patient was incapacitated, his or her surrogates had to initiate the discussion of whether to remove the respirator. The whole thrust of this policy was to protect the hospital against law suits by lessening the possibility that the question of whether to remove a respirator would arise. Misplaced concern about legal liability appears to have outpaced concern about the well-being of the patient on the part of the institution and its administrators.

The *Guidelines* recommend that all patients, but especially those with serious or terminal illness, such as Tony, be given opportunities to discuss their condition and future options with caregivers and to make decisions about the kind of treatment that they want. [*See* Part One: "Making Treatment Decisions," II., (2) "Evaluation and discussion"; (3) "Identifying the key decisionmaker"; and (4) "Making the decision."] This does not mean that massive doses of information should be foisted onto patients at the moment of diagnosis or that they should be forced to make all decisions regarding future treatments at that point. Instead, patients should be allowed to learn about their illness, prognosis, and treatment alternatives at a pace that seems appropriate to them individually. Under ideal circumstances, this would involve a series of conversations with physicians and other health care professionals that lead to the development of a treatment plan. In such a plan, the immediate and long-range goals of treatment are outlined, and a decision tree is developed that sketches the series of treatments that will be adopted, each depending on the outcome of preceding treatment, as far into the future as it is feasible to plan. It is useful to put such a plan in writing, so that all present and future caregivers will be aware of it.

A treatment plan for patients who face critical illness will also take into account the possibility that the patient will lose decisionmaking capacity temporarily or permanently during the course of the illness. To provide for this circumstance, patients may wish to attach a treatment directive to their treatment plan or to their medical records in which they outline the kind of treatment that they would want should they enter a certain condition or conditions and become incapable of making their own decisions. [*See* Part Three: "Prospective Planning; Advance Directives."] Critically ill patients who are at serious risk of death should be encouraged to develop treatment plans with their primary caregiver and to make decisions about the use of life-sustaining treatment and surrogates as early in the course of their illness as they can. In doing so, they should be advised that their condition may change and that their current choices are not irrevocable.

Advance directives represent the basic moral choices of patients who develop them and should be adhered to by those caring for them. There may be occasions when physicians and nurses have good reason to think that a patient has been grossly misinformed in developing a treatment plan or an advance directive or when the patient's prognosis changes radically and unexpectedly from that anticipated in the plan and immediate emergency action must be taken that conflicts with it. In such cases, the plan or directive should be set aside only if discussions are initiated with the patient or surrogate immediately afterward. It is my belief that such instances will be rare.

Part Four

Declaring Death

19. Crossing Over:
The Case of Mrs. Larson

Wilma Larson, a seventy-eight-year-old woman, was admitted to County Medical Center after she suddenly collapsed downtown. Resuscitative efforts in the ambulance and the Emergency Room restored a normal heart rhythm, but she was deeply comatose with evidence of severe brain damage. Soon after her admission, her daughter came into the ER and demanded to see her mother. Mrs. Larson was undergoing intensive medical therapy in the ER at that time and could not be seen. Her daughter became very upset and hostile.

Mrs. Larson was admitted to the Coronary Care Unit of County. On the second hospital day, she was deeply comatose with unstable vital signs. She was maintained on a respirator and given medications to support her blood pressure. The family was told that an EEG would be obtained that day to determine the degree of brain damage she had incurred. Later that day, however, the family was informed that Mrs. Larson was moribund, that death would occur at any time, and that an EEG was unnecessary. They were angry about receiving this contradictory information from hospital personnel.

On the third hospital day, Mrs. Larson was still critically ill and deeply comatose, but she had not expired. Her family was irate because the medical staff continued resuscitative efforts for her. The family unanimously requested that these efforts be discontinued and that their mother be allowed to die.

Mrs. Larson's immediate family consisted of her husband, four children, and numerous grandchildren. They revealed that in the few weeks before her collapse, Mrs. Larson had experienced a premonition that she was going to die. She had made out her will, calmly discussed death with her husband and the rest of the family, and made numerous other arrangements—she even had dinner downtown with all of her old friends. Her family strongly believed that death would be welcomed by her at this time. Her children expressed the belief that their mother should be allowed to die; they had strong religious convictions about life after death. Mr. Larson, who had a dementing illness, did not take an active part in the discussions.

At least two of the children had been very aggressive and hostile throughout the three days of Mrs. Larson's hospitalization, and this had created numerous conflicts between them and the hospital staff. At the end of the third day, a son and two grandchildren took up guard over her to prevent any further nursing or medical care. The nurses and several of the medical staff in the Coronary Care Unit felt that these relatives were interfering with the provision of care that they had a professional duty to give.

A neurological examination was done at this time. It revealed that Mrs. Larson was deeply comatose with fixed, dilated pupils, no spontaneous respirations, and no clinical evidence of cortical or brain stem activity. The neurological consultant found that she had demonstrated no evidence of brain activity for over twenty-four hours.

There was considerable discussion at this time among members of the medical and nursing staff about how much longer resuscitative efforts should be continued. Everyone agreed that Mrs. Larson's prognosis for conscious existence was virtually zero. There was also a discussion of who should make the final decision. Some felt that it was the family's right to decide whether to stop resuscitation; others felt that it was the responsibility of a CCU physician.

What should be done for Mrs. Larson at this time? Who should decide? Has she received appropriate care up to this point?

Commentary by Ronald E. Cranford

This case and the ethical problems it presents must be placed in perspective. This clinical dilemma is based on an actual case that occurred in the early 1970s when these physicians did not have a great deal of experience in diagnosing brain death and were not comfortable about pronouncing individuals dead using neurologic criteria. There were no state or national criteria for the medical determination of brain death other than the 1968 Harvard criteria at that time. There was no Uniform Determination of Death Act, and only a handful of states had enacted legislation.

The section on the declaration of death in the *Guidelines* [see Part Four: "Declaring Death"] represents a distillation of the knowledge and wisdom that we have accumulated since then. Now, in the mid-1980s, this patient would have been taken care of in significantly different ways at this institution. Thus, it will be useful to show how Mrs. Larson would have been treated today to demonstrate the importance of developing guidelines and evolving a medical and social consensus on determining death. This issue is far less controversial and unsettled than many other issues covered in the *Guidelines*.

The first few hours of Mrs. Larson's hospitalization would not be handled any differently today than they were then (nor should they be). Because this was a true cardiorespiratory emergency, the medical staff still would initiate maximal therapeutic measures in the Emergency Room and in the first few hours in the Intensive Care Unit. The physicians did not and would not know enough about the values and preferences of Mrs. Larson to be justified in ceasing resuscitative efforts on her behalf in this emergency situation. The Emergency Room is not the setting in which to evaluate a patient's lifestyle, her premonition of death, her saying "good-bye" to everyone, and the feelings of her family. The initial phase of Mrs. Larson's hospitalization illustrates an increasingly common dilemma: the medical staff initiates appropriate emergency care, but when this is viewed from the perspective of the patient and family, this was not what the patient would have wanted, was not in her best interests, and was not in the best interests of the family.

Today, however, the physicians would "shift gears" much sooner than they did in this case. They would be much more experienced and competent in determining brain death and pronouncing death. The medical criteria at this facility, recommended by the institutional ethics committee, are the standards established by the consultants to the President's Commission for the Study of Ethical Problems in Medicine of 1981—which were also endorsed by the state medical association in early 1982. At the present time, an observation time of six hours combined with a radio-isotope blood flow study (not an EEG, which was abandoned years ago at this facility) would have been adequate to diagnose brain death. The family would have been spared the anguish and grief of the futile prolongation of life for a period of several days after the physicians had informed them of the utterly hopeless prognosis.

This case, therefore, illustrates how continually refining and improving the medical criteria for diagnosing brain death while retaining the basic definition of death, using cardiorespiratory and neurological standards (irreversible cessation of all functions of the entire brain, including the brain stem), can decrease the possibility of administering futile treatment and the inadvertent creation of family suffering. The state in which the case occurred is one of the few remaining states without a statute or a state supreme court decision on the validity of brain death as a standard of death. However, in the majority of cases of brain death at this institution and throughout the state, the standard of practice is to pronounce patients dead using neurological criteria.

According to almost every statute and court decision and every national medical standard for brain death, once a person is determined to be brain dead, he or she is dead and pronouncement of death is mandatory. Consent of the family is medically and legally irrelevant and, in theory, the views of the family should have no bearing on the determination of death. However, it has been the unofficial policy at this institution not to pronounce the patient dead or to discontinue life-support systems until the medical staff has addressed any *reasonable* concerns, questions, or objections the family may have.

(It should be noted that at this institution the delay in the final pronouncement of death and the discontinuation of life-support systems have no bearing on the actual time of death—which is the time at which the absence of all brain functions was first noted, i.e., at the beginning of the period of observation.)

The physicians informed Mrs. Larson's family of her utterly hopeless prognosis, but then seemed hesitant to stop treatment—let alone pronounce the patient dead. The family was literally standing guard over this patient at the bedside, preventing further nursing and medical care in the Coronary Care Unit. What should happen when the concerns of the family are not deemed reasonable by the medical staff or when there is an obvious conflict of opinions, as in Mrs. Larson's case?

If a parent wants to continue treatment on his brain dead child when the parent is alleged to have caused the child's present condition, then our practice and the guidelines would make the course of action clear. The child would be pronounced dead using essentially the same criteria and procedures for determining death as in other circumstances—over the objections of the parent because of the obvious conflict of interest. If the family continued to object, a referral to the hospital ethics committee would be suggested or the family could seek legal counsel and try to obtain a restraining order preventing the health care providers from declaring death. This is the policy that would be followed for Mrs. Larson as well. It appears that many physicians, however, are not comfortable in diagnosing death and that many, in conflicts like this, would temporize and wait for the vital signs of heart beat and respirations to disappear as the patient developed more medical complications.

Brain death is death, and society (as well as the *Guidelines*) has accepted the view that the pronouncement of death and the discontinuance of life-support systems is mandatory—except in certain well-delineated circumstances, as when treatment is continued in a patient for the purpose of maintaining organs for donation and in a brain dead mother when there is a potential for delivering a viable fetus. While society places great value on pluralism and individual religious views, the determination of death, as opposed to the forgoing of medical treatment in patients who are critically ill but not brain dead, must be applied in a uniform way.

The ethical dilemmas in this particular case were resolved with the help of the ethics committee, which suggested further neurologic evaluation to clarify whether Mrs. Larson was brain dead. [*See* Part Five: "Policy Considerations," Section A. "Ethics Committees."] This condition was substantiated by further neurological consultation. Life-support systems were discontinued after the patient was pronounced dead, using the neurological standard.

20. The Long Dying:
The Case of "Flip" Harrow

STUNTMAN "FLIP" HARROW DECLARED BRAIN DEAD

Los Angeles, December 12 {Sunday}—This morning at 10:03 AM Los Angeles born and bred stuntman, "Flip" Harrow, fell 500 feet to the ground after his parachute failed to open during a jump for the filming of the movie *Space Race*. Harrow suffered severe brain and spinal cord injuries.

Tonight he is hovering near death and is listed in critical condition in the intensive care unit of Hollywood Heights Hospital. His brain damage was compounded by the fact that Harrow went without breathing for some time as rescuers combed the area for him.

Los Angeles Detective Samantha Clark said she arrived at the crash site fifteen minutes after the accident occurred. "He was more or less all mangled up beneath a tree," said Clark. She said that after Harrow was put onto a stretcher, his heart stopped beating, and CPR was administered.

Referring to Harrow's parents who were called in London, Linda Seaver, nursing supervisor at the hospital said, "They were absolutely devastated."

Hollywood physician, Earl Grey, who treated Harrow at the site of the accident, said that if Harrow's situation does not improve, the family will have to decide how long to leave him on the respirator.

"He's a person who loves life," movie director Oscar Steinberg said of Harrow.

Los Angeles, December 13 {Monday}—The injuries to Harrow left the stuntman brain dead. With cardiac stimulants and fluid replacement to keep his blood pressure up, Harrow was still alive tonight, but was given no chance to survive.

"We will now work with the family to decide how far they want to go in sustaining his biological life," said Dr. Sara Evans, one of the doctors treating Harrow. Without a respirator, Evans added, Harrow would stop breathing "in a matter of minutes".

Grey said the respirator keeping Harrow alive would be disconnected "as soon as the family can deal with the idea. . . . I'm concerned about the mother's health, too. She's not well. I understand she has a significant heart condition."

Los Angeles, December 14 {Tuesday}—"Flip" Harrow, the Los Angeles stunt-man who has been brain dead since he fell 500 feet from a Cessna airplane early Sunday morning, was declared dead tonight after surgeons removed all of his vital organs for possible transplantation.

Harrow, 35, who suffered extensive brain and spinal injuries, was officially declared clinically dead Monday morning while his heart and lungs were kept functioning by a respirator.

Lisa Davies, who plays the part of "Angel Diver," the character for whom Harrow performed the stunt, said, "If his organs can be donated, that will help others and 'Flip' will live on."

When did "Flip" Harrow die? Why is this question at issue?

Commentary by Robert M. Veatch

The report of stuntman "Flip" Harrow dying comes from a press release or newspaper story, so it is hard to determine who is responsible for the confusion that it contains. Regardless of who is responsible, it presents some terrible issues of conceptualization as well as problematic moral choices.

The first task is to get clear when Harrow died and on what grounds he should be called dead. The report on Monday describes him as "brain dead," but also says he is "still alive." The writer of the story (and perhaps the clinicians who provided the information for the story) must have held that people can be alive, even though their brains have "died." This displays serious misunderstanding of what it means to be dead in California. There is a legal definition of death in California that requires that "a person shall be pronounced dead if it is determined by a physician that the person has suffered a total and irreversible cessation of brain function." A similar statute or similar case law defines death as the total cessation of total brain function in almost all jurisdictions in the United States. Whether or not we agree with the moral and philosophical judgments inherent in that stipulation of what it means to be dead, that is the law. Harrow should have been called dead at the time that it was determined that his brain had irreversibly lost all its function.

The term "brain death" is systematically ambiguous. It now normally means that the person as a whole is to be treated as dead for legal purposes based on the irreversible loss of brain function. That is not a scientific judgment, even if it is one about which there is an increasing consensus. The term can also be used in another sense, however. It can refer to the death of the brain in someone who is still considered to be alive. Those who use the term in this fashion would have to believe that it is possible to be considered alive even though one has a dead brain.

It would make sense to refer to someone as "living with a dead brain" in a jurisdiction that has not authorized the pronouncement of death based on brain criteria (as of 1987, the states of Delaware, Minnesota, South Dakota, and Utah), but technically one cannot be alive with a dead brain in those jurisdictions that require death to be pronounced in such situations. Thus, the writer of this story, in implying that Harrow is alive with a dead brain, is either confused about the jurisdiction or is purposely taking exception to California law.

The story gets more confusing when we read that Harrow was declared dead on Tuesday after surgeons had removed all his vital organs for possible transplantation. To make matters worse, Harrow was also "declared clinically dead" on Monday. It is almost impossible to imagine what being "clinically dead" means if it does not refer to the irreversible stopping of either the brain or the heart and lung function. Some people erroneously consider people to be dead "temporarily" if heart and lung function stop in a way that can be reversed. Being dead is, by definition, an irreversible phenomenon. One cannot die temporarily.

Because of all these confusions it would be better if the terms "brain dead" and "clinically dead" were abandoned. We should talk about Harrow and others as either dead or alive. One could also add that they are considered dead based on brain or heart and lung criteria, depending on the jurisdiction or the philosophical convictions of the speaker.

That death was pronounced after the removal of Harrow's "vital" organs poses an even more serious moral problem. It implies that he was not only considered dead based on heart and lung criteria, but also that the physicians were the ones who caused the death. If Harrow was, in fact, pronounced dead after the heart was removed, this is good evidence that it was the clinicians who were confused and not the writer of the story.

There is some evidence that we should be concerned about whether Harrow's brain function was really irreversibly lost. Dr. Sara Evans states that he would "stop breathing in a matter of minutes" if the respirator were disconnected. A person without any brain function would not breathe at all after a ventilator was disconnected. He would not breathe for minutes. What is described appears to be more like an individual who has irreversibly lost all higher brain functions, but retains some brain stem activity. Such a person is not dead, even according to laws in jurisdictions that have adopted brain criteria for pronouncing death.

Some philosophers and other commentators have taken the position that even individuals who retain lower brain functions (such as respiratory regulation) should be considered dead. They hold that a person no longer exists "as-a-whole" because some essential element of the person is irreversibly lost. There is no scientific argument against that position. It is really not a scientific question. Nevertheless, no state has adopted the view that persons are dead when they lose higher brain function.

The story also seems confused when it states that "if Harrow's situation does not improve, the family will have to decide how long to leave him on the respirator." Several issues are raised here. Assuming that Harrow really is dead because his brain is dead, we are dealing with a respiring corpse. Technically it is correct to say at this point that the family could have a role in deciding how long Harrow remains on a respirator. Although he is dead, a decision could be made to maintain the corpse for worthwhile purposes including use of organs for research, teaching, transplantation, or other therapeutic purposes. If organs are to be maintained, however, permission is needed according to the law governing the use of anatomical organs and tissues. Harrow's own wishes, if expressed while competent, are governing. The physicians could (and many believe should) maintain his organs even against the wishes of the family if Harrow had executed a document making a Uniform Anatomical Gift Act donation. If he had not, however, his next-of-kin must agree.

If, on the other hand Harrow is not dead, but merely seriously injured and dying, then the judgment about continued life-support should be governed by Harrow's own wishes if they are known. If they are not known, many people hold that the family's or surrogate's wishes should be decisive unless they are proved to be malicious or unreasonable. It is conceivable that the family or surrogate could therefore decide to remove him from a ventilator even if he improves somewhat. On the other hand, they might insist that the respirator continue even if he does not improve.

Physician Earl Grey, if quoted correctly, seems to believe that physicians have the discretion to continue ventilation and to continue to treat Harrow as alive in order to give the family time to adjust to his demise. If Harrow's brain is destroyed, he cannot be made alive by the physician's desire to permit the family to adjust. Physicians have no such discretion under current law. It is conceivable that they could pronounce death but fail to tell the family in order to give them time to adjust. Such a course raises moral problems about truth-telling but would at least follow the legal requirement that death be pronounced. Since next-of-kin permission is needed to preserve the corpse for use of organs (assuming Harrow himself had not agreed in advance), a strategy of failing to tell the family would presumably also be one of forgoing the opportunity to preserve the organs.

Finally, we understand what Lisa Davies means when she says that Harrow can "live on" if his organs are donated. In some symbolic way that may be true, but it is extremely important to realize that Harrow is really dead— dead all the way—when brain function ceases irreversibly. He does not live on in any legal or philosophical sense.

Under current California law, Harrow should have been pronounced dead at the time that irreversible loss of total brain function was confirmed. Assuming Harrow had not made a donation under the Uniform Anatomical Gift Act, the family should have been asked for permission to maintain the body for transplantation purposes. If he was not really dead based on loss of all brain function, the family should have been asked whether they wanted ventilation stopped so he could die.

The *Guidelines* [*see* Part Four: "Declaring Death"] adopt the standard of the Uniform Determination of Death Act, which requires cessation of the entire brain for a declaration of death. I am convinced, however, that the higher brain function concept of death is more reasonable than a "whole-brain-oriented" concept of death. I would like to make it possible for persons who have lost higher brain function irreversibly to be declared dead. On the other hand, I realize many do not share this view. Out of respect for the plurality of ethical and religious convictions in the United States, I believe that the default position of the law should be that persons are declared dead when all brain function ceases unless they have opted for a higher brain or a heart and lung concept of death or, if they have not expressed their views on the subject, their next-of-kin opts for an alternative definition of death on their behalf.

Part Five

Policy Considerations

21. By What Authority?
The Case of Mario Costanza

A man fell to the ground in a shopping mall and did not respond to the queries of passersby. One of them called an ambulance that took him to the Emergency Room of a nearby hospital. There he was placed on a respirator and was diagnosed as having suffered a brain stem infarction that had permanently destroyed spontaneous respiration and cardiac function. At this time, he was identified by a nurse who knew him from several previous admissions as Mario Costanza, a sixty-nine-year-old man.

Mr. Costanza was moved to a bed in the Intensive Care Unit of the hospital. During the course of his care, he would respond to painful stimuli by withdrawing. He would move his eyes to follow an object upon request. Although he seemed to try to talk, he could not utter any sound. He appeared to respond to questions at times by nodding his head. He alternated between long periods in which he seemed to be in a "vegetative" state and short periods in which he seemed to be minimally conscious.

When his wife asked him whether he wanted all treatment ended, Mr. Costanza made no effort to answer. She thereupon authorized a "No Code" order in the event that her husband's heart stopped functioning and requested that all other forms of aggressive treatment cease, including the use of the respirator. She said that she and her husband had carried on long conversations about what he would want done if he should ever enter a condition such as this and that he had clearly indicated that he would not want heroic treatment.

Mr. Costanza's doctor, however, adamantly refused to put the "No Code" order into effect or to discontinue treatment for him, for he said that he was not sure that the patient was in a persistent vegetative state. He kept Mr. Costanza on the respirator, provided suctioning for his tracheostomy, and maintained a nasogastric tube for feeding. He said that he would provide any other treatment that was necessary to keep Mr. Costanza alive, despite the wishes of his wife.

Mr. Costanza's son agreed with his mother that this treatment was futile and that his father would not want it. Mr. Costanza's current nurses, who had spoken with nurses who knew him from his previous admissions, began to think that continued aggressive treatment was contrary to wishes that he had expressed earlier. They spoke to the hospital chaplain who, in turn, spoke to Mr. Costanza's physician. The physician still refused to withdraw aggressive treatment / The chaplain, who was chair of the hospital's ethics committee, determined that there was sufficient concern among the staff and the patient's family to convene a meeting of the hospital ethics committee.

When the chaplain told Mr. Costanza's physician of the upcoming meeting of the ethics committee, the physician became very angry. He wanted to know by what authority the nurses and chaplain were challenging his orders. He was a powerful figure in the hospital, he said, and he would speak to the chief of the medical staff to have the hospital ethics committee disbanded. He refused to attend the committee meeting.

Does a hospital ethics committee have the authority to act in a situation such as this? Should it meet without the physician? If it does, what sort of action should it take?

Commentary by Cynthia B. Cohen

A motivating force behind the original formation of hospital ethics committees was the desire of health care professionals to resolve some of the pressing ethical questions raised by their developing power to sustain life. Early ethics committees served as confidential groups in which perplexing ethical issues could be discussed among health care professionals as they arose in specific cases. As these committees made progress in advising about difficult cases and in facilitating interprofessional communication, they began to provide consultations not only to health care professionals, but to patients and their families. Eventually, it was realized that the experience and knowledge that they were gaining could be used to assist in the development of policies and educational programs for the entire institution. Historically, therefore, the early ethics committees evolved from serving as advisory groups to health care professionals to functioning as patient counselors and institutional advisory bodies on policy, as well. This concerned some conscientious physicians who came to think, as the functions of ethics committees grew, that they had inadvertently created a monster in the hospital ethics committee with the potential to destroy the physician-patient relationship.

Mr. Costanza's physician is evidently one of these health care professionals. That he is not adept at handling threats to his professional autonomy, however, does not indicate that his concern about the involvement of the ethics committee in Mr. Costanza's case is unfounded or irrational. Health care professionals realize that the face of medicine is changing and that a variety of forces are impinging on the traditional physician-patient dyad, including ethics committees. They are also aware that, as yet, no dependable means for evaluating how well these committees are functioning have been devised. Anecdotes drift through operating rooms and physicians' lounges of the damage that these committees do, as well as of their usefulness in advising about difficult cases and defusing interprofessional and professional-patient conflicts. It is not surprising, therefore, that opinion is split among health care professionals about the value of these committees and that some physicians refuse to meet with them.

Whether this ethics committee has the authority to override the objections of Mr. Costanza's physician and to consider Mr. Costanza's situation without the approval of his physician depends on why and by whom the committee was established and what institutional and state rules and regulations govern it. The institution has a responsibility to ensure that good decisionmaking procedures are being followed for its patients. If the ethics committee was developed, in part, to assist in meeting this responsibility and was consequently empowered to serve as an advisory unit to health care professionals and to patients and their surrogates, then it probably can consider Mr. Costanza's case without the approval of his physician. Health care professionals who are involved in Mr. Costanza's treatment have asked for an ethics consultation on his case from the committee, and it is implied that his wife and son are also interested in having the committee meet. The basic requirements for convening a meeting of an advisory hospital committee therefore appear to be met.

Although the committee can meet when the patient's primary physician refuses to have any contact with it, can it function without him? It is important that ethics committees learn about the diagnoses and prognoses of patients whose care they review from qualified medical professionals, for good ethical decisions are based on good medical information and judgment. The fact that this information will not be supplied to the committee by Mr. Costanza's physician, however, is not a barrier to review in this case, for the information can be developed from other sources. (Should there be a question of patient confidentiality, the consent of Mr. Costanza's wife, his apparent surrogate, for access to medical information about him should be sought.) However, the absence of the primary physician at an ethics committee discussion of a patient's situation can mean that special insights into the wishes of the patient are lost, for the primary physician may have been uniquely apprised by the patient of these. Since Mr. Costanza was unable to communicate effectively with others from the time of his admission, and does not appear to have been known by the physician from his previous admissions, his current physician could not have exclusive information about his values and beliefs. The committee, therefore, need not rely solely on the physician either for medical evaluation or for an indication of the patient's wishes in this case.

The major thrust of the committee's deliberations should be to recommend a range of ethically acceptable options for Mr. Costanza's care that would be in his interests at this time. These interests are determined, in part, by his current medical prognosis and, since he cannot currently express himself, by his previously expressed wishes and values. We have limited information about Mr. Costanza's medical prognosis. It is not clear that he is in a permanently vegetative condition, for he tracks with his eyes and may be reacting to pain purposively. It does appear that any decision to maintain somatic life will involve the use of a respirator for as long as that decision stands. It is vitally important that Mr. Costanza's condition be confirmed by experts in neurology before the committee meets. Once the diagnosis and prognosis are established with reasonable probability, the committee must then consider the patient's wishes and values in order to make a recommendation.

Since Mr. Costanza cannot communicate, a surrogate decisionmaker must be found for him. There is no reason to believe that his wife is not an acceptable surrogate. Her statements about what her husband would want done should be taken seriously, although care must be given to ensure that once his diagnosis is confirmed, she understands it and fits his previously expressed wishes to it. The nurses who have known Mr. Costanza from earlier admissions also appear to be reliable witnesses concerning his previous treatment preferences and values. If their information and that of the son, as well, confirms that Mr. Costanza would not want to be maintained by a panoply of medical technology in his current condition, it would be appropriate for the committee to recommend that aggressive treatment for him be ended and that supportive care be instituted instead. However, care must be taken to ensure that his current condition *is* the condition that he had in mind when he said that he would not want heroic treatment.

To whom would the committee make its recommendations? To a physician who is hostile to the group and who has refused to cooperate with it. If the committee is effectively to meet its goal of recommending what it considers to be in the interests of patients, it must also address the concerns of the medical staff who are treating these patients. Even if the committee is authorized to function by the institution's governance, and perhaps even required to do so by state law, accrediting bodies, or third party insurers, whether it can act successfully is highly dependent on the support of health care professionals who practice at the institution. The threat of Mr. Costanza's physician to destroy the committee should not be dismissed lightly. A strong figure within the hospital could impede the committee to a point where it became useless.

To avoid these problems and to attempt to achieve what is beneficial for Mr. Costanza, the committee could designate a member or two who know the physician to talk with him and learn of his concerns. Ideally, this would be done before the committee enters the final stages of its deliberations, so that the physician does not feel that he is presented with a *fait accompli* that he cannot influence. A way that is sometimes effective in bringing an opposing health care professional to a committee meeting is to explain to the individual that the committee needs to take his or her opposition into account and to learn from it. Even those who firmly object to the functioning of ethics committees can play an important role in their improvement, for they have valuable criticisms that such committees need to consider. A committee member or members appointed to reach Mr. Costanza's physician who take this tack with him might be able to alleviate his fear and hostility toward the group and to bring him to the meeting.

The *Guidelines* recommend that when a patient lacks the capacity to make a treatment decision, a surrogate should be identified who "is most involved with the patient and most knowledgeable about the patient's present and past feelings and preferences" to decide for the patient. [*See* Part One: "Making Treatment Decisions," II., (3) "Identifying the key decision-maker," (b) "Identifying a surrogate."] The obvious surrogate for Mr. Costanza, according to the *Guidelines* and on the basis of information we are given in the case, is his wife. The surrogate is to act in accordance with the patient's wishes when these are known or else as a reasonable person in the patient's circumstances would. [*See* Part One, II., (4) "Making the decision," (c) "The patient who lacks decisionmaking capacity."] If Mr. Costanza's wife is choosing on the basis of accurate medical information and seems to understand his previously expressed preferences correctly, there is good reason to respect her decision on her husband's behalf. If, however, she is choosing on the basis of a misunderstanding and refuses to reconsider her decision, further steps will have to be taken to address the problem.

The *Guidelines* recommend consultation with institutional ethics committees that review ongoing cases when there are ethical issues to be resolved. [*See* Part Five: "Policy Considerations," Section A. "Ethics Committees."] If the ethics committee concluded that Mrs. Costanza did not understand her husband's diagnosis and prognosis or was misinterpreting his wishes, it could recommend to the hospital administration that legal action be initiated to protect Mr. Costanza if she persists in authorizing the withdrawal of treatment from her husband. If, on the other hand, the committee concluded that the physician is mistaken about Mr. Costanza's prognosis and/or that Mr. Costanza would not want to receive all available life-sustaining treatment in his current condition, as his wife maintains, it could recommend a transfer of Mr. Costanza's care to another physician. [*See* Part One, II., (1) "Underlying ethical values," (c) "The ethical integrity of health care professionals."]

22. Too Terrible to Accept:
The Case of Maisie Wedmore

Maisie Wedmore, an eighteen-year-old, had a cardiac arrest following back surgery. She was diagnosed as having severe hypoxic encephalopathy (severe brain damage caused by lack of oxygen) as a consequence and was placed on a respirator. She also suffered permanent damage to her kidneys during the arrest, and dialysis was begun. One month later, she was diagnosed as being in a persistent vegetative state. Although she did not respond to verbal stimuli in any way, she did react to loud auditory stimuli with a startle response. At that time, she could breathe without the assistance of a respirator and had sleep-wake cycles.

After repeated neurologic examinations by different physicians, it was concluded that Maisie's condition was irreversible. This poor prognosis was fully explained to her parents. Mrs. Wedmore did not seem to comprehend or to accept these explanations and said that she was sure that her daughter would recover. She wanted maximal treatment for Maisie, including intensive care, full resuscitation status, and a kidney transplant. Maisie's father wanted all treatment for her ended. The parents were divorced; they had retained joint custody of Maisie until her eighteenth birthday.

Maisie's physician and the chaplain have talked with Mrs. Wedmore on numerous occasions and have tried to explain the hopelessness of her daughter's condition to her. Nurses, too, have tried to help her come to terms with her daughter's state. Mrs. Wedmore, however, has been unwilling to accept the diagnosis. Indeed, she avoids discussions of it when she can. This situation has lasted for three months.

The physicians are very troubled by the case and refer it to the hospital ethics committee.

Is this an appropriate case for referral to an ethics committee? If so, what procedures should the committee follow in addressing the problem? If not, what should be done instead?

Commentary by Ronald E. Cranford

Ethics committees have been established in recent years to assist health care professionals, patients, and families in dealing with, and it is hoped, in resolving dilemmas such as those presented by Maisie Wedmore's case. How could an experienced and knowledgeable ethics committee have been of value to Maisie, her parents, and the health care professionals caring for her?

An ethics committee's functions, as outlined in the *Guidelines* [*see* Part Five: "Policy Considerations," Section A. "Ethics Committees"], are basically four: education, policy formulation, consultation, and prospective review. Assuming that this ethics committee has been in place for several years, the health care professionals at the institution would know of its existence and of its advisory role through its previous educational and policy-formulating activities. They would also know that requests for committee consultations are optional and that committee recommendations are not binding.

This committee might well have had educational programs for staff on individual wards or for the entire hospital staff on the current moral-legal status of the treatment of patients such as Maisie who are in a persistent vegetative state. It would have discussed issues such as how to minimize conflicts between families of such patients and health care professionals, how to try to resolve their differences in the institutional setting, how cost containment policies affect their choices, and the role that economic considerations should play in these decisions. As the committee gained experience, stature, and credibility, it may have made its members available informally for questions from health care providers ("curbside consults"). If the ethics committee is large and has representatives from most major wards of the hospital, health care professionals might have felt free to discuss matters informally with the ethics committee representative on their ward. The ethics committee would also have developed a mechanism for handling more formal consults, as discussed in the *Guidelines*.

An experienced ethics committee would have recognized that Maisie's case presents a difficult ethical dilemma for which there is no easy solution. There appears to be a genuine conflict of values in this case that makes it a paradigm of ethical dilemmas that we will increasingly face in the future. A primary question that it presents is what should an ethics committee do when it learns that a health care professional, patient, or family is clearly acting outside the range of what seems morally and medically permissible? How long could the health care professionals at this institution, or the ethics committee in its advisory role, permit continued acute care hospitalization and intensive care for a patient in a persistent vegetative state? How far should health care providers go in acquiescing to the wishes—or the "unreasonable demands"—of Mrs. Wedmore? Who determines what is "unreasonable"? How much effort should be made to help Mrs. Wedmore understand and appreciate the hopeless nature of her daughter's condition?

There are three things that ethics committees almost invariably do when they are involved with specific cases: (1) Establish that the medical facts are correct. (Is this patient truly in a vegetative state? Would a kidney transplant be medically indicated?) (2) Stress the importance of communication and facilitate communication in various ways. (Why does the mother feel this way if the prognosis is truly hopeless? Has every reasonable attempt been made to understand the mother's views? Have there been adequate care conferences in which all those involved discussed the case from medical, moral, and legal standpoints?) (3) Identify the central issues, conflicts, and ethical dilemmas and, as in this case, recognize the extreme difficulty of finding an adequate resolution. (What should health care professionals do when a primary decisionmaker, such as the mother, adamantly refuses to discuss the issues? What impact will the continued care of this patient have on other patients and health care professionals?)

A properly constituted ethics committee that represents multiple disciplines and views of the hospital and the community could be expected to provide a broad spectrum of opinions on these matters. If there were a strong consensus on the committee that it would be wrong to continue acute care for Maisie after a reasonable period and that it would be wrong to do a kidney transplant, this would carry a great weight. On the other hand, if there were a great deal of disagreement among the members of the ethics committee, this would reflect a great divergence within the institution and community and would indicate that no one decision is clearly appropriate. This is one reason why we have ethics committees rather than individual ethics consultants alone. It seems reasonable that a large number of people would more accurately represent the views of the institution and the community than would one individual.

In this case, the health care professionals and ethics committees should do everything reasonably possible to be as honest and frank with the family as they can be, even though Maisie's situation is hopeless. They should be extremely attentive and sensitive to the needs and views of family members and the complex dynamics of family relationships.

The committee could offer specific ways that cases like this have been handled and resolved in the past; in this respect ethics committees act in a quasi-judicial manner, building on previous case precedents. The ethics committee could also point out to caregivers, based upon its reading of the literature and its experience, that it may take months or years before family members can fully emotionally and intellectually accept the diagnosis of persistent vegetative state and the hopeless prognosis. It is invariably difficult for the family to accept the possibility that non-treatment may be the most appropriate course of action. In the vast majority of cases, however, families are quite reasonable and, with adequate time and discussion, will reach a satisfactory solu-

sonable and, with adequate time and discussion, will reach a satisfactory solution.

The *Guidelines* emphasize that conflicts should be resolved intra-institutionally whenever possible, with court review only as a last resort, and that institutions should establish some mechanism for dealing with ethical disputes and conflicts. In the majority of cases, the ethics committee serves this invaluable role, and there is no need for involvement of the courts. However, this is one case in which the ethics committee might need to recommend court action. This would especially be the case if the mother continued to demand continued care that would have a negative impact on other patients.

Many committees have already formulated policies on Do-Not-Resuscitate orders and brain death in the last ten years. In the near future, these committees will develop policies addressing the management of patients in the persistent vegetative state and other severely ill or disabled patients—policies that would have helped in this case. Ethics committees will assess strengths and weaknesses of such guidelines as they are put into practice, modify them according to institutional or local needs, recommend their adoption to the appropriate hospital authorities, be responsible for their dissemination and for staff education about them, and be available for questions on their implementation.

23. No Place Else to Go:
The Case of Ernest Brown

Six months ago, Ernest Brown, a sixty-year-old man, was diagnosed as having metastatic cancer of unknown primary origin. No surgery, chemotherapy, or radiation therapy were expected to offer cure or palliation. Since the time of his diagnosis, his cancer has gradually become more extensive, and over the past three weeks, Mr. Brown has become weaker; he is unable to eat more than one-half bowl of rice and soup a day. He has become jaundiced, and his abdomen and legs have become more and more swollen.

Mr. Brown and his family understand that his prognosis is grave. His family consists of a son, daughter-in-law, and three young grandchildren. When he was first diagnosed, his son said that he wanted to care for his father at home. However, Mr. Brown's recent deterioration has been especially difficult for his daughter-in-law to manage, and his son has brought him to the Emergency Room of the local hospital.

Evaluation in the Emergency Room reveals a weak, malnourished man with end-stage cancer and signs of possible sepsis and peritonitis. He has a prognosis of only days to weeks. Blood tests, including blood cultures, are drawn, and an IV is begun.

Mr. Brown's son tells the Emergency Room physician that he had tried to get his father into a publicly funded nursing home or a hospice program, but that his father did not qualify because he was his son's dependent, and the son was considered to have an adequate income to provide for his care. He cannot afford to have him cared for in a private nursing home, however, and he has reached the end of his emotional and financial resources in caring for him at home. He has to think of his wife and three children, too. He tells the physician that he wants his father to be comfortable and well cared for—and then he leaves the hospital. Mr. Brown is admitted to the Medical Service.

What can and should be done for Mr. Brown now? What could and should have been done for him earlier?

Commentary by Joanne Lynn

Mr. Brown's situation is a serious indictment of a health care system gone awry. Key components of care for a dying person include access to symptom control, continuity of care, support and encouragement from caregivers, care that addresses the needs of the patient's family, and appropriate attention to advance directives. None of these is evident in Mr. Brown's care.

The most obvious shortcoming in his care prior to this last hospitalization is that he and his family should have been offered adequate supportive services which would have allowed him to stay at home without unbearable burdens. Most likely, this would have included at first only weekly visits by a nurse or a social worker to assess those needs that were becoming evident and to ensure that all understood the medical situation and the plans. Later, as he became more disabled, planned periods of respite for Mr. Brown's daughter-in-law provided by someone who came to the home to care for him (perhaps for three hours twice a week) would probably have become essential to everyone's mental health. As he developed specific self-care deficits, such as being unable to bathe himself, a home health aide who came to do this service, perhaps every other day at first and every day as he became worse, would have spelled the difference between all concerned feeling good about the care provided for Mr. Brown or feeling overwhelmed and inadequate.

Throughout this period, a physician should have seen the patient as needed and at least once a month. It is essential to evaluate whether any of the problems that develop are treatable and to ascertain that advance directives about future care are as clear and comprehensive as possible [see Part Three: "Prospective Planning; Advance Directives"] and that the care provided by others is meeting the patient's needs adequately. It is worth noting that a fatal cancer such as Mr. Brown's that causes fluid in the abdomen and jaundice is likely to cause death by hepatic failure. Somnolence is the major evident component of such failure and frequent physician assessments are not likely to be necessary.

Most families that receive this sort of support will feel comfortable about having the patient die at home. A competent nurse or physician will need to be available to such a family at all times and will need to be able to come to the home to assess any changes in symptoms or to help with emotional and administrative concerns at the time of death. The case as presented does not provide the ages of the children involved or their responses, but it is very likely that it will be better for their long-term mental health to have Mr. Brown die at home than to go off to die in a hospital where they cannot visit and where they can imagine all sorts of terrible things happening.

Our current systems of health care routinely do not insure for this sort of care and ordinarily do not have home care and care of the dying organized so as to serve actual needs. Nevertheless, Mr. Brown and his family probably could have benefitted greatly from competent legal and financial help. Would his care options actually improve if he were not considered his son's dependent, for example? Removing him from his son's tax reporting is usually a simple thing to do. Charging him some rent and applying for Medicaid may qualify him for various services, depending upon the rules of each jurisdiction. No explanation is given as to why a man so young (only sixty years old) is his son's dependent. If it is because he is disabled, he may be eligible for Medicare, which would make him eligible for paid hospice services.

Of course, all of this is "water under the bridge" when he comes in to the Emergency Room. [See Part Five: "Policy Considerations," Section B. "Institutional policies for patient admission and transfers," III. "Hospitals," (4) "Emergency Rooms."] Nevertheless, the ER physician should try to assess whether any clear plans have been made about the care at the end of life before starting treatment for an illness that is not particularly uncomfortable and might rapidly be fatal. In this tense and emotional situation, though, the ER physician is not likely to be able to forgo life-extending treatment on the basis of unclear or newly formulated statements of what is to be done. The medical situation is likely to be somewhat unclear and the emotional situation for father and son is certain to include guilt, remorse, self-blame, anger, and fear. A decision at this time to allow the elder Mr. Brown to die will be uncomfortable for both of them.

Nevertheless, the decisions to treat and to admit can be made in as supportive a way as possible. The son can be reassured that he is not unworthy or inadequate for being worn out and that his concerns for his family are appropriate. He also can be encouraged to think of this admission as a possible opportunity to recover from emotional exhaustion, so as to be more able to be responsive to the needs of his father if he survives this episode and to the needs of himself and his family in any case.

If the elder Mr. Brown is mentally clear, his views on his own care should obviously be solicited and plans made to clarify them over the next few days. Since he may lose mental clarity, it is important that someone talk with him, someone who knows the actual extent of supportive services for which he may be eligible. Of course, the fact that he may feel that he has just been put out of home will have to be kept in mind. If he is not forceful in stating a desire to have no life-extending treatment or if the medical situation is not one in which the forgoing of life-sustaining treatment is virtually the only appropriate option, one would be uncomfortable in failing to treat his problems acutely. However, treatments at this stage can and ordinarily should be set up as time-limited trials, both to establish how well he will respond and to allow time for him to formulate a coherent care plan guiding his future care.

Irrespective of what else is done, the patient deserves treatment for symptoms. Probably the tense fluid in the abdomen and legs could be relieved with removal of some of the fluid or with medications. As additional symptoms develop, they will need careful assessment and treatment. Most of the symptoms and disabilities of dying cancer patients develop in the final few weeks of life.

It will be harder to arrange home care now than it would have been to provide adequate care for Mr. Brown throughout his prior course. His caregiving family is now exhausted, and there is no agency that has been involved and is now willing to stretch some to accommodate extensive care needs. Home care hospice programs might be able to help, but he apparently has no funding and will have to rely upon charity for this sort of service. [*See* Part Five: "Policy Considerations," Section B. "Institutional policies for patient admissions and transfers," V. "Hospices."] Discharge to a nursing home is likely to be thought undesirable on all sides: the patient is likely to find this depressing, the son would likely find it financially and emotionally devastating, and the nursing home would not have enough time to work with the patient to shape a better life before he became too ill to benefit and died.

Such a patient is difficult for a nursing home setting, as much for his impact upon staff and other residents as for the difficulties of adequate symptom relief. [*See* Part Five: "Policy Considerations," Section B. "Institutional policies for patient admissions and transfers," IV. "Nursing Homes."] The physician in the hospital should ensure adequate follow-up and might actually arrange an informal plan for periodic respite admissions for Mr. Brown so as to make home care more possible for his troubled family.

Thus, if Mr. Brown's condition stabilizes and he seems to have at least a few weeks left, his discharge planning will be difficult and his entire future may be spent in a hospital that does not wish to serve him and will not be paid for the services provided. Having Mr. Brown die comfortably and having his family feel good about their role may yet be possible, but it is going to take much more work on the part of those into whose care he has now been delivered than it would have taken if adequate care had been provided all along. One can hope that institutions and providers that repeatedly see this sort of situation will become advocates for better care systems and more responsive ways of funding them.

24. Trapped in "the System": The Case of Sam Jones

The Emergency Room physician was told by the nursing home administrator that they were sending a sixty-seven-year-old man over to the hospital because he had mild shortness of breath and they just wanted to "play it safe." The patient, Sam Jones, had lived in the city-managed nursing home for the past two years. He had been admitted from the public hospital, where he had been diagnosed as having chronic obstructive pulmonary disease.

At one time, Mr. Jones had operated a passenger elevator in a local department store, but for the ten years before his admission to the nursing home, he had lived essentially as a "street person." His only known relatives were two nephews who had little do with him. Once he was settled at the nursing home, Mr. Jones expressed interest in his surroundings and chatted amiably with other residents.

Mr. Jones had been transferred to the hospital Emergency Room frequently during the past two years for treatment of his respiratory difficulties. During recent talks with his primary nurse, he said that he no longer wanted to be sent to the hospital, that he did not wish to be placed on life-support machines, and that he would prefer to die in the nursing home among friends. However, no orders to this effect were written in his treatment plan. The nursing home was poorly staffed and was currently operating under provisional licensure for uncorrected medical and nursing citations. This latest transfer of Mr. Jones to the Emergency Room was authorized by a night nurse who was unfamiliar with his wishes.

Mr. Jones was awake, alert, and oriented on his arrival at the hospital. He was given oxygen and medication, which improved his respiratory symptoms, but the ER physician, who had never seen him before, felt that he needed to be admitted to the ICU. Mr. Jones said that he wanted to be sent back to the nursing home and did not wish to go to the ICU. He asked the admitting doctor to call his nurse at the home.

The ER physician called and told the charge nurse that Mr. Jones would die if he returned to the nursing home. She told the physician of Mr. Jones's repeated requests to die in the nursing home and of his desire not to be placed on a respirator. She said that she hoped that just because he was poor, his wishes would not be disregarded. The nursing home administrator told the physician that they were willing to take Mr. Jones back, but only on the condition that he had improved, as the facility was no longer prepared to care for patients with severe respiratory illnesses.

The ER physician then contacted Mr. Jones's physician of record. The physician said that he was not sure of who Mr. Jones was and that he would defer to the ER physician's judgment. Repeated efforts to contact Mr. Jones's two nephews were unsuccessful.

After Mr. Jones had been in the Emergency Room for five hours, he was admitted to the ICU. On his third night in the ICU, he experienced increasing difficulty in breathing, and the resident on call ordered intubation and mechanical ventilation. Two weeks after he entered the ICU, Mr. Jones died there.

Did Mr. Jones receive appropriate treatment? If not, what should have been done for him instead?

Commentary by Mathy Mezey

The ethical dilemmas raised by this case are three-fold: (1) What obligations do health professionals who gather information about patients' wishes have to ensure that such wishes are respected? (2) How can health professionals protect patient autonomy as people move across a health care system that is frequently fragmented and uncoordinated? (3) How can we ascertain whether patients are placed in appropriate health care institutions that are capable of providing services in conformity with their needs and stated preferences?

The primary nurse caring for Mr. Jones knew of his expressed wishes not to be placed on life support and to die in the nursing home. We are unclear, however, as to what actions the nurse took to assure that Mr. Jones's wishes were followed. Were his wishes conveyed to the primary physician or the Director of Nursing in the nursing home? Were they documented in the hospital record? It is not unusual for a patient such as Mr. Jones to be assigned a physician in the hospital with no prior knowledge of his medical condition. Similarly, it is not uncommon for the nursing home physician of record to be unfamiliar with a patient's prior personal or medical conditions and not be the physician of record on a subsequent hospitalization. Frequently a primary nurse is the professional who has the most continuous contact with a patient who is repeatedly hospitalized with symptoms such as those of Mr. Jones. This nurse is also the professional most familiar with the patient's preferences concerning a treatment plan. In the nursing home, in all likelihood, it is the nursing staff who have primary responsibility as a matter of fact for Mr. Jones's medical management.

In the absence of written orders stating Mr. Jones's preferences concerning transfer and medical care in either the hospital or nursing home records, it is unlikely that the physicians who are unfamiliar with Mr. Jones will feel comfortable in offering anything but full treatment on each hospital admission. When physicians or nurses on the scene are unsure about the depth of a patient's conviction regarding a preference to withhold treatment, the principles of beneficence (doing good) and maleficence (not inflicting harm or evil) come into direct conflict with, and frequently supersede, a desire to preserve patient autonomy. Yet, by virtue of law and custom, the nurse, who is the professional most familiar with the patient's desires and wishes, is frequently precluded from documenting these preferences and writing orders in the hospital record.

According to the American Nurses' Association Code of Ethics, nurses have a responsibility to promote patient autonomy and to assure that patients' decisions are appropriately supported. At the very least, it is the nurse's responsibility to document Mr. Jones's preference in the hospital record, to discuss Mr. Jones's preferences with his responsible health care professional, and to contact the nursing home administration about them. If such discussions and actions prove unsatisfactory, or if the responsible health care professional feels unsure about his or her responsibility regarding Mr. Jones's treatment decisions, this ethical dilemma can appropriately be brought to the institutional ethics committee. [*See* Part Five: "Policy Considerations," Section A. "Ethics Committees."]

The question of how to assure adherence to patients' treatment decisions as they move from one institution to another remains extremely problematic. The lack of familiarity of the responsible health care physician in the nursing home with Mr. Jones's medical condition or his preferences is not atypical. Because of distance or inconvenience, nursing home admission frequently necessitates that a patient be assigned a new physician who is unfamiliar with the patient's past medical and social history. Following the admission history and physician examination, regulations and reimbursement place severe limitations on subsequent physician visits to patients in nursing homes. These factors partially explain the fact that primary care physicians spend less than 1.5 hours per month in nursing homes.

The *Guidelines* recognize that in nursing homes and in home care, registered nurses at times assume the role of responsible health care professional *de facto*. In Mr. Jones's case, if the Director of Nursing or another professional nurse had been designated to do so, it would have been his or her responsibility to ensure that Mr. Jones's treatment decisions were appropriately followed. Given that the nursing home was poorly staffed and acting under a provisional license, it is unlikely that the nursing staff, no matter how well intentioned, could have made a case to the administration for keeping Mr.

Jones in the home in his debilitated state. Medicaid and Medicare reimbursement provide disincentives to keeping such patients in nursing homes and serve instead to promote hospitalization. Moreover, the nursing care Mr. Jones required might have detracted from the staff's ability to care for other patients, thereby raising issues of justice.

What is lacking in this case is the clear emergence of either a physician or a nurse who is in charge of Mr. Jones's care as he is moved between nursing home and hospital. Failure to designate a responsible health care professional who can supervise the course of care irrespective of a patient's place of residence, and failure on the part of hospitals and nursing homes to require that such a professional be appointed, relegates patients such as Mr. Jones to a state of limbo when trying to assure compliance with their treatment decisions.

The third issue is how to ensure that patients such as Mr. Jones are placed in institutions that are capable of rendering care commensurate with their medical condition and their stated treatment preferences. For long stay patients such as Mr. Jones, it is not unusual for medical conditions and treatment preferences to change over the course of a nursing home stay, which may span several years. Mr. Jones's initial medical needs and treatment preferences may have been well matched to the nursing home's capabilities when he was originally admitted. However, as the case suggests, both Mr. Jones's treatment preferences and the nursing home's ability to render care have changed over time. In fact, at the time we meet Mr. Jones, the nursing home is unable and unwilling to care for him or to comply with his desires to avoid future hospital transfers. Whose responsibility is it to assure that Mr. Jones is placed appropriately? Is it reasonable to expect that, given his medical and economic condition, Mr. Jones can negotiate his own best placement? What is the responsibility of the physician, of the nurse, of the two institutions involved in Mr. Jones's care, and of the state and federal government who are paying for his care?

The *Guidelines* offer suggestions as to the need to match patient characteristics with institutional capabilities and indicate circumstances under which patients should not be admitted, discharged, and transferred. [*See* Part Five: "Policy Considerations," Section B. "Institutional policies for patient admissions and transfers," IV. "Nursing Homes."] The processes for implementing such recommendations, however, are left primarily to the good will of the participating parties. It is imperative that institutions establish mechanisms to facilitate implementation of these recommendations.

25. The Costs of Addiction:
The Case of Rita Anderson

Rita Anderson, who is forty-two years old, is addicted to drugs and alcohol. She has attempted to overcome her dependencies in five different in-patient drug treatment programs without success. Her parents, who have tried to help her, have finally disowned her from the large family estate. Because she is unable to support or care for her twelve-year-old daughter, the girl has lived with Ms. Anderson's parents for the past ten years.

Ms. Anderson is now in severe heart failure and is a patient at Community Hospital. She has received one prosthetic heart valve, but needs and wants a second due to reinfection. Her physicians at Community recommend the heart surgery for her. However, because of her frequent hospitalizations, she has reached the $1 million lifetime maximum coverage provided by her medical insurance policy, and she does not have the means to cover the cost of the operation. Community Hospital will neither accept Medicaid, nor consider doing open heart surgery for Ms. Anderson without payment.

Arrangements are being made to transfer Ms. Anderson to County Hospital, where Medicaid funds will cover most of the costs of her surgery. The physicians at County, though, are reluctant to admit her. They feel that while the surgical risk in her case is good, it would be futile to replace the valve, since there is a strong chance that Ms. Anderson will resume behavior that will lead to reinfection. In addition, they are convinced that Ms. Anderson will not follow the prescribed drug regimen after surgery. Finally, County Hospital does not have the resources to cover the extra costs of the surgery that are not reimbursed by Medicaid.

Should the surgery be provided, since Ms. Anderson wants it? If so, how should its costs be covered?

Commentary by Robert M. Veatch

Two basic ethical questions are raised by this case. First, can care ever be prohibited because of social or economic costs involved, and second, if so, can the voluntary behavior of the patient that leads to the need for the care ever provide reason for prohibiting it?

First, there can be no doubt that in some cases the social and economic costs of providing care are a legitimate basis for exclusion of care. The total amount of care that people desire—including cosmetic interventions, intensive private psychotherapy, and extremely expensive long-shot trials of therapy that is unlikely to work—might well exceed the gross national product, even if we limit calculations to the United States. If care desired by all people in the world were considered, it would surely exceed the resources that are available. Some care must be limited on socio-economic grounds.

There are three moral bases for setting such limits. Some would permit people to buy (or to buy insurance for) whatever medical services they desire, provided they can afford it. Under this principle, if Ms. Anderson cannot pay for her surgery and has exhausted her insurance coverage, she should be turned away unless someone wants to give her the care as an act of charity.

Others would advocate the use of health insurance dollars on the basis of which investments of these dollars would do the most good overall. It is an empirical question whether investing in Ms. Anderson's second chance would do more good than investing similar health insurance resources in someone else's care. It would also depend on whether the good taken into account was so-called "medical good," which would include increases in life-expectancy and decreases in morbidity, or whether the good under consideration was social good as well.

Many people object to such calculations on the grounds that they are unfair. They particularly object to the consideration of non-medical goods when deciding about whether to provide medical treatment. Others reject even policies that attempt to maximize medical good. This position is taken by people who are committed to egalitarian theories of justice, according to which people are to be given opportunities to be as healthy as other people—even if the total amount of medical good done is not as great as it otherwise could be.

The third strategy, the egalitarian strategy, would ask not how much good treatment would do for Ms. Anderson in comparison with other patients, but rather who has the greatest claim in equity for the care. This approach raises additional issues. If the resources are not given to Ms. Anderson, who would benefit from the alternative use of them? Even if Ms. Anderson is in greater need than other patients who might benefit from the resources, should she receive a second opportunity to be as well as others?

That leads to the second major question: can the voluntary behavior of a patient be the reason for prohibiting care? Introducing this issue in Ms. Anderson's case will require some empirical judgments. In particular, is Ms. Anderson's drug and alcohol abuse a voluntary behavior? If it is not, then we cannot exclude care for her on grounds that she must accept the foreseeable consequences of her voluntary behavior. Deciding whether behaviors that create risks to health are voluntary can be extremely difficult. Many behaviors may be determined by biological, genetic, psychological, or social causes beyond the individual's control. According to various analysts, Ms. Anderson may be addicted because of a gene for alcoholism, socio-economic factors, or her toilet training.

Assuming that her behavior is voluntary, is that a basis for cutting off care for her? It would be if she is entitled only to an opportunity to get what she needs and she has squandered that opportunity. However, even if this were the case, society might still provide care for her because there is simply no way to cut it off without generating unacceptable social impacts. In some cases, we would not want to bar people from hospitals who are in need of treatment in order to survive because it would make others in society too uncomfortable. In other cases, the purportedly voluntary behavior might not have an established correlation with the health risk. In still other cases, the risky behavior might be worthy of societal support. We would not exclude people who work in socially worthwhile but risky professions like firefighting from health care simply because they voluntarily take chances.

Abusing drugs and alcohol are hardly worthwhile social endeavors that are deserving of public support. They may be difficult to monitor, however. One strategy that has received increasing support is to identify behaviors that are detrimental to health and that can be monitored and to place a fee on them that reimburses insurance funds for the marginal health costs of engaging in such behavior. We might put a health fee on the use of ski lifts, for example for they are easily monitored, seem to be voluntary, and are probably not worthy of public subsidy in the way that firefighting is.

The most likely reasons to oppose limiting care for Ms. Anderson are that her choices may not be voluntary and that, even if they are, it is not clear that society could tolerate leaving her to die without care.

If some care must be limited, we will need to determine how such decisions ought to be made and what the role of clinicians ought to be in making those choices. Some would have the clinicians, in this case the clinicians at Community Hospital, decide whether Ms. Anderson is entitled to the expensive care. This would involve them in socio-ethical judgments that have nothing to do with medicine. They would have to decide whether care should go to those with greatest need or to those for whom it can do the most good. They would have to decide whether the resources could better be used for other health care or even for goals outside of health care. Physicians ought not to make such judgments because they tend to have unusual values. They naturally place special importance on health care, so it is likely that they would overcommit society's resources to this area. Even if they did not place atypically high value on prosthetic heart valve replacement, they would have to decide what the role of voluntary health risk ought to be. Since this is a non-medical judgment, many people have concluded that clinicians ought not to be the ones making decisions that limit medical care on socio-economic grounds. [*See* Part Five: "Policy Considerations," Section C. "The use of economic considerations in decisions concerning life-sustaining treatments."]

Even more fundamentally, clinicians have traditionally had as their moral duty the service of the patient. Under the Hippocratic ethic they were to do what they thought was for the benefit of the patient. Today, many people prefer that they serve the rights of the patient, including the right of the patient to refuse treatment, rather than opting for paternalistic definitions of patient welfare. Nevertheless, these people hold that clinicians ought to remain patient-centered. If that is the case, making decisions to limit care on socioeconomic grounds is incompatible with the moral mandate of the health care professions.

If care must be limited, and it cannot be limited by the clinician, someone else must set its boundaries. One scheme that seems to make sense is to ask the lay population to make these decisions. If they were asked to determine what services should be covered in order for coverage to be fair to everyone in society, the result could be a fair insurance system. It would give priority to patients for medical care on the basis of ability to pay, the amount of good the care would do, or the need of the patient, depending on the ethical stance taken by society.

Regardless of which stance is taken, some limits would be built into the insurance system. This would be true whether it were a private insurance system or, as many believe is morally preferable, a publicly funded insurance program. Once the coverage for certain forms of medical care was excluded, the administrators of the system would have a duty to make sure that no patient had access to such care under insurance funding, even if clinicians believed that the care would be beneficial for the particular patient.

The lay population could plausibly insist that voluntary risks should be funded by means of special health fees on the behaviors involved where such fees were paid into the insurance system to cover the extra margin of care. While risks resulting from illegal behaviors (such as drug use) could not be funded in this manner, those resulting from legal behaviors could be. Excessive alcohol consumption is so clearly risky not only to the imbibers, but to others as well, that a good case can be made that its use ought to be made illegal. If it remains legal, alcohol consumption should have a fee attached to it that is calculated to equal the marginal health care costs involved. If the care for Ms. Anderson were funded in this matter, then there would be no problem in providing her with the care that she needs in order to survive. If the care is not so funded, then society ought to consider adopting insurance standards that do not permit expensive services for such behaviors if they are deemed voluntary.

26. When is Patient Care Not Costworthy? The Case of Gertrude Handel

The following dialogue occurred during Grand Rounds:

Dr. Kittredge: Gertrude Handel, a sixty-year-old woman, has had cancer of the pancreas for six months. The cancer has metastasized despite her participation in an experimental chemotherapy program. Currently, 95 percent of her liver is cancerous, she has metastases in her lungs, and her peritoneal cavity is filled with malignant ascites [cancerous fluid]. The patient has become anuric [her kidneys have stopped functioning], and she is encephalopathic [has suffered severe brain damage] due to kidney and liver failure.

The family has been told that she is dying and that there is nothing further that medical science can do for her. They have been advised that the present aim should be to keep the patient free from pain and as comfortable as possible. However, the family refuses to accept this and insists on placing the patient in the Intensive Care Unit to receive all available aggressive treatment.

I would like to begin our discussion by asking Dr. Sakabe whether there is a possibility that the prognosis for this patient is more favorable than was indicated to the family.

Dr. Sakabe: The prognosis seems quite accurate. Intensive care would prolong the patient's life for a few days at most. The patient has no chance of recovering from the brain damage. Further, this is a particularly unresponsive form of cancer. Studies indicate that those who have it, even those who have participated in experimental protocols, invariably die. I do not think that the family has been misinformed.

Dr. Kittredge: What is the current bed situation in the ICU, Dr. Sakabe?

Dr. Sakabe: The beds in the ICU are all occupied. I have asked whether there is any other patient who could be safely discharged to make room for the patient, but there is none.

Dr. Kittredge: Are there any other ICUs at nearby hospitals that could treat Mrs. Handel?

Dr. Sakabe: I have called around to see what we might be able to arrange; but no other ICU in the community is willing to admit the patient.

Dr. Kittredge: Dr. Bernstein, have you spoken with the family about the patient's wishes?

Dr. Bernstein: Yes, I have. They say that the patient has told them on several occasions that she would want everything possible done to keep her alive if she should ever become terminally ill.

Dr. Kittredge: Did you discuss the costs of intensive care for the patient with them?

Dr. Bernstein: No, I didn't. The patient has catastrophic health care insurance, and the effect of the costs of her care would not be felt by the family. It seemed the wrong time to bring up costs with them, as they were very upset, and the costs do not directly affect them.

This seems to me to be a major problem, though. Shouldn't we consider the costs of intensive care? Although the expenses incurred by additional treatment won't financially devastate the patient and her family, they *do* affect the costs of medical care to others who are in the patient's insurance pool. This has been overlooked by patients and physicians and is one reason why the costs of medical care have been rising so rapidly. Another reason is that we don't stop to consider whether some of the medical care we are providing is worth its high cost—or whether it is wasteful or useless. Some expensive medical treatments should be carried out, it seems to me, because they can restore patients to a meaningful life. But in this case, further treatments cannot do that. They would be futile, and it seems wrong to ask others to pay for them.

Dr. Kittredge: Dr. Lean, would you also comment on the question of the expense of providing intensive care for this patient?

Dr. Lean: While I have a great deal of respect for Dr. Bernstein's opinions, I believe that he is way off base if he thinks that doctors should consider the costs of care that they provide to patients. It is essential to the ethic of medicine that physicians ignore costs. Once we begin to talk about whether money should be spent on some patients and not others, we get into a devilish kind of reasoning that ends in allowing elderly people to die because their care is too expensive and that dumps poor people out of ERs because they have no insurance coverage. No one has a right to put a price on a patient's life. I know that I could never consider how much money each procedure costs when making a treatment decision for my patients. It would be contrary to everything that I stand for as a doctor.

Dr. Kittredge: What would you do in this case, then, Dr. Lean?

Dr. Lean: Well, I must admit that I, too, am bothered by the idea of giving the patient treatment that will only keep her alive for a few more days at great expense. I just want someone else, not me, to decide when treatment is too costly to provide. We shouldn't make these kinds of decisions at the bedside. We need some kind of policy that we know is ethical for determining when treatment is just not worth its costs.

Dr. Kittredge: The question of how to contain the costs of medical care presents one of the most intractable problems that modern medicine has to face. The two different points of view that you have presented here indicate that poli-

cies need to be developed by responsible persons or bodies to contain the rising costs of medical care in ways that are ethical and fair. We have to face
the fact that some patients and their families will be denied their preferences
for certain kinds of treatment because that treatment is too expensive and ineffective.

In this case, it seems to me that we should tell the family—as gently
as possible—that we cannot provide the treatment that they want because
there is currently no room in the ICU. We are not the appropriate group to
talk about the costs of intensive care with them, especially at this point in
their lives. It is not our responsibility to determine who will live and who
will die on the basis of how expensive their treatment is.

But we cannot just impose this news on the family and then walk
away. We need to sit down with them and help them to talk about their painful situation. This is a time when we especially need the help of the chaplain, hospice nurses, and social workers. It won't be easy, but we have no
other choice.

Should Mrs. Handel be denied admission to the ICU because her care
would not be costworthy? If so, should her family be apprised of this?

Commentary by Dan W. Brock

The central issue raised by this case is what role, if any, physicians should
play in rationing health care when benefits seem not worth its costs. More spe-
cifically, should Mrs. Handel's physicians make decisions "at the bedside"
about whether particular health care for her is worth its cost? It is easy to sym-
pathize with Dr. Bernstein's concern about the social bill for expensive care
such as that which Mrs. Handel's family seeks for her, since it appears to be
both wasteful and inappropriate. At the same time, it is also easy to sympa-
thize with Dr. Lean's concern that if physicians ever begin to decide whether
care for their patients is worth its cost, they will inevitably be carried down
a slippery slope toward clearly wrongful denials of care to the old or poor.
Any plausible response for limiting use of noncostworthy care must be sensitive to both these concerns.

It is sometimes said that for so important a good as health care, cost
should never be a consideration in whether a particular patient receives it. I believe it is easy to see that this cannot be correct. There is wide agreement
that it is ethically permissible for a competent patient to decide to forgo any
life-sustaining care that he or she judges to be unduly burdensome. One of

the burdens of care is the financial cost that it imposes on the patient or others about whom the patient cares. Patient resources used for health care will not be available for other uses. Thus, a patient might freely choose not to undergo some forms of even life-sustaining treatment in order, for example, to preserve an inheritance for his family. Few would find such a choice based on consideration of financial costs ethically objectionable.

When a patient is incompetent to make treatment choices for him or herself, a surrogate, commonly a family member who knows the patient best, must decide for the patient. The widely accepted substituted judgment principle requires that surrogates attempt to decide as the patient would have decided in the circumstances if he or she had capacity. If there is clear and compelling evidence that the patient would not have wanted a particular treatment, in part because of its expense, respecting the patient's self-determination strongly supports the decision of the patient's surrogate against the costly care. Thus, there is nothing intrinsically unethical in either patients or their surrogates sometimes deciding to forgo treatment because of its cost.

The specific issue this case raises, however, is whether Mrs. Handel's physicians should take it upon themselves to deny care to her that she and her surrogates want solely on grounds that its benefits do not warrant its costs. I believe there are several important reasons why they should not. First, Mrs. Handel has obtained catastrophic health care insurance presumably in order to be able to pay the costs of care in circumstances like these. While this does not obligate her physicians to offer whatever care her surrogates might demand for her, it probably does obligate them not to deny her care on grounds of its cost. Her insurance, in effect, creates both an entitlement and a legitimate expectation that any medically appropriate care covered by her policy will be paid for by the insurance. While the insurance payments for her care will come from the pooled funds largely of others, all members of a private insurance pool join together to pool their funds precisely in order to fund members' entitlements to reimbursement for catastrophic health care costs. Even if the insurance comes from a government program funded by general tax revenues, that program would have the same democratic legitimacy as would other government spending programs, and the entitlements the program establishes should be honored, not surreptitiously undermined, by Mrs. Handel's physicians.

Institutions such as the government, employers, and health insurers all have an interest in holding down their bill for health care. They should not expect or pressure physicians, however, to deny care to patients in circumstances like Mrs. Handel's in which patients have an entitlement to be reimbursed for the financial costs of care. That would be to put the physicians in an ethically unacceptable position. It *is* ethically acceptable for physicians to help patients or their surrogates weigh the true costs of care against its benefits when the patients or surrogates wish to do so. I believe it is also ethically acceptable for the incentive structures of reimbursement systems to encourage patients or surrogates to weigh the true costs of care against its benefits more than is now common, so long as that does not result in denying patients an adequate level of care. The main reason this is so notoriously difficult to do is that health care insurance, the means of reimbursement for most health care in our country today, reduces or eliminates both out-of-pocket costs to the patient for care utilized, and in turn, the patient's economic incentive to consider or even learn the true costs of care. Yet the unpredictability and great variability in the amount and cost of health care that an individual may need provide powerful reasons to have insurance for health care costs.

A second important reason why Mrs. Handel's physicians should not take it upon themselves to decide whether her care is too costly to the other members of her insurance pool is that they lack any social, moral, or legal authorization to do so. If there is to be a serious public debate in this country about limiting utilization of noncostworthy care, particularly if that is life-sustaining care, then we are now only in the early stages of that debate. Any authorization for physicians to act as health care rationers with their individual patients should come as a result of such a debate, and not merely from pressures from third party payors to reduce their health care outlays. These pressures would be likely to fall most heavily on the vulnerable and powerless and would perhaps end up realizing Dr. Lean's worst fears.

When cost containment measures are openly adopted in financially closed health care systems like HMO's, then both physicians and patients can have reasonable assurance that cost savings will be passed on in the form of lower rates, improved quality of care, or new available forms of care to members who have forgone care to produce the savings. In such settings, it is possible for patients and physicians to cooperate together with the shared goal of providing good quality health care while limiting health care costs. When physicians instead only reduce "society's" overall health care costs by denying care that may benefit or be wanted by their patients, their justification cannot be that the savings are returned to those denied the care for them to spend in alternative ways.

A third serious concern about physicians assuming the role of health care rationers with their individual patients is whether denials of noncostworthy care would be equitably or fairly applied to different patients. If physicians are left to determine without further guidance what care is costworthy for individual patients at the bedside, then almost certainly the effects of these attempts to control health care costs will *not* be equitable. This is because physicians, in the absence of clear standards of costworthy care, would inevitably reach differing conclusions about what care is costworthy and would also be susceptible to allowing ethically irrelevant factors, such as the social worth of the patient, subtly to influence their judgments. The relatively vulnerable and powerless could be expected to suffer a disproportionate share of the effects of such rationing.

A fourth major concern about physicians becoming "bedside rationers" is that this will create new conflicts of interest between patients and their physicians and so be likely to undermine the trust necessary for well-functioning physician/patient relationships. If physicians come to think of themselves as responsible for ensuring that society's resources are prudently spent, patients' trust that the treatment recommendations and decisions of their physicians are guided first and foremost by concern for their patients' well-being will quite justifiably erode. I think that this concern lies behind Dr. Lean's view that physicians should remain unconstrained advocates for their patients and that "someone else . . . should decide when treatment is too costly to provide."

These various worries about physicians becoming bedside rationers do not imply that economic considerations should never play any role in decisions concerning life-sustaining treatment. Instead, they support an ethical case: (1) that decisions about standards and/or procedures for identifying care that will not be provided to patients because it is not costworthy be arrived at through public processes that allow substantial input to those who will be affected; (2) that health care institutions limiting access to noncostworthy care inform current and potential patients of those limitations; (3) that procedures be put in place to monitor the application of limitations on provision of noncostworthy care to insure that it is done equitably and without denying patients access at least to an adequate level of health care.

The appropriate decisionmaking bodies for defining limitations on noncostworthy care will vary depending on the context. For example, in an HMO these issues might be addressed by a committee within the HMO with substantial patient member representation. For government insurance programs, open debate at relevant points in the political process such as legislatures, public hearings, and so forth, would be appropriate. In other cases, participant input may be fostered by employers and health insurers that provide their employees and insurees with a greater range of alternative insurance plans that attempt to define and limit reimbursement for noncostworthy care to varying extents. There is no single institutional mechanism or group of persons that should address and make decisions about what care is costworthy. Nor is there any single correct definition of costworthy care, or any ethical necessity for societal uniformity in the definitions arrived at.

These several reasons for Mrs. Handel's physicians not to deny her the aggressive care she seems to have wanted because it is too costly do not mean she must go to the ICU. Because there is no available ICU bed, Dr. Kittredge is right that the family should be told, as gently as possible, that the treatment they want cannot be provided because there is no room in the ICU.

Even if an ICU bed is available, the hospital may have a policy, such as the *Guidelines* recommend [*See* Part Five: "Policy Considerations," Section B. "Institutional policies concerning patient admissions and transfers," III. "Hospitals," (5) "Intensive care units," (a) "Admissions," (3)], that patients with irreversible organ system failure be admitted to the ICU only if they cannot be treated appropriately in another setting. If this is the established and explicit policy of the hospital, made known to patients (and/or their families) early in their hospital stay, then Mrs. Handel's physicians should explain that, and why her transfer to the ICU is not appropriate. If no agreement can be reached about the patient's care, they should offer to withdraw from the case and to help the family facilitate transfer of the patient's care to another institution.

Dr. Bernstein characterizes the aggressive life-sustaining measures the family seeks as "futile." Certainly, most people would not want them for themselves or their loved ones. Dr. Sakabe concedes, nevertheless, that they might extend Mrs. Handel's life by a few days, and the evidence suggests that both she and her family consider that a desirable benefit. Denial of care on grounds of "medical futility" should be reserved for those treatments known definitely to have no chance of prolonging life. They should not be used to hide physicians' value judgments that the benefits produced are too limited to warrant their use. This case illustrates that when treatments are characterized as futile for the latter reason, patients or surrogates may not share the value judgments that the label of "futility" conceals.

The *Guidelines* on the use of economic considerations in decisions concerning life-sustaining treatments are less detailed and specific in their recommendations than are the rest of the *Guidelines* because there is no well-developed public or professional consensus in this area that the *Guidelines* might articulate. [*See* Part Five: "Policy Considerations," Section C. "The use of economic considerations in decisions concerning life-sustaining treatments."] Nevertheless, the *Guidelines* do address the problem faced by Mrs. Handel's physicians in stating that health care professionals should not cut costs or ration medical resources except in accordance with patient wishes or explicit institutional or governmental policy. If either of these conditions is satisfied in Mrs. Handel's case, the *Guidelines* do not support having her physicians deny care that her surrogates indicate that she would want on the grounds of cost. In this respect, the *Guidelines* tell her physicians what *not* to do.

I believe the *Guidelines* are at least as important in their positive recommendations in support of the kind of public dialogue that I have suggested above about how to define and whether to limit noncostworthy care. The *Guidelines* quite correctly note that there is nothing inherently unethical in the use of economic considerations in decisionmaking about life-sustaining treatment and call for a public policy process that could result in ethically defensible determinations and limitations of noncostworthy care.

BIBLIOGRAPHY

General Readings

HEALTH CARE ETHICS

Beauchamp, Tom L., and James F. Childress. *Principles of Biomedical Ethics*, 2d ed. New York: Oxford University Press, 1983.

Beauchamp, Tom L., and Laurence B. McCullough. *Medical Ethics: The Moral Responsibilities of Physicians*. Englewood Cliffs, NJ: Prentice-Hall, 1984.

Benjamin, Martin, and Joy Curtis. *Ethics in Nursing*. 2d ed. New York: Oxford University Press, 1986.

Callahan, Daniel. *Setting Limits: Medical Goals in an Aging Society*. New York: Simon and Schuster, 1987.

Gorovitz, S., R. Macklin, A.L. Jameton, J.M. O'Connor, and S. Sherwin, eds. *Moral Problems in Medicine*, 2d ed. Englewood Cliffs, NJ: Prentice-Hall, 1983.

Hunt, R., and J. Arras, eds. *Ethical Issues in Modern Medicine*, 2d ed. Palo Alto: Mayfield, 1983.

Jakobovitz, I. *Jewish Medical Ethics*, 2d ed. New York: Block Publishing, 1975.

Jameton, Andrew. *Nursing Practice: The Ethical Issues*. Englewood Cliffs, NJ: Prentice-Hall, 1984.

Oden, Thomas C. *Should Treatment Be Terminated? Moral Guidelines for Christian Families and Pastors*. New York: Harper and Row, 1976.

O'Rourke, Kevin D., and Dennis Bordeur. *Medical Ethics: Common Ground for Understanding*. St. Louis: The Catholic Health Association of the United States, 1986.

President's Commission for the Study of Ethical Problems in Medicine and Biomedical and Behavioral Research. *Deciding to Forego Life-Sustaining Treatment*. Washington, DC: U.S. Government Printing Office, 1983.

Shelp, Earl E., ed. *Virtue and Medicine: Explorations in the Character of Medicine*. Boston: D. Reidel, 1985.

Thompson, Joyce B., and Henry O. Thompson. *Ethics in Nursing*. New York: Macmillan, 1981.

U.S. Congress, Office of Technology Assessment. *Life-Sustaining Technologies and the Elderly*. Washington, DC: U.S. Government Printing Office, 1987.

Veatch, Robert M., ed. *Life Span: Values and Life-Extending Technologies*. New York: Harper and Row, 1979.

Weir, Robert F., ed. *Ethical Issues in Death and Dying*, 2d ed. New York: Columbia University Press, 1986.

LEGAL OVERVIEWS

Cantor, Norman L. *Legal Frontiers of Death and Dying*. Bloomington: Indiana University Press, 1987.

Doudera, A. Edward, and J. Douglas Peters, eds. *Legal and Ethical Aspects of Treating Critically and Terminally Ill Patients*. Ann Arbor, MI: Health Administration Press, 1982.

Robertson, John A. *The Rights of the Critically Ill*. Cambridge: Ballinger Press, 1983.

Society for the Right to Die. *The Physician and the Hopelessly Ill Patient: Legal, Medical, and Ethical Guidelines*. New York: Society for the Right to Die, 1984.

TEACHING HEALTH CARE ETHICS

Ackerman, Terrence F., *et al.*, eds. *Clinical Medical Ethics: Exploration and Assessment*. Lanham, MD: University Press of America, 1987.

Culver, Charles, *et al.* "Basic Curricular Goals in Medical Ethics," *New England Journal of Medicine* 312 (1985):253-256.

Davis, Anne J. "Ethics Rounds with Intensive Care Nurses." *Nursing Clinics of North America* 14 (1979):45-55.

Dickinson, G. E. "Death Education in U.S. Medical Schools: 1975-1980." *Journal of Medical Education* 56 (1981):111-14.

Dietrich, M. C. "A Proposed Curriculum on Death and Dying for the Allied Health Student." *Journal of Allied Health* 9 (1980):25-32.

Eichna, L. "A Medical School Curriculum for the 1980s." *New England Journal of Medicine* 308 (1983):18-21.

Elkins, Thomas E., Carson Strong, and P.V. Dilts. "Teaching of Bioethics within a Residency Program in Obstetrics and Gynecology." *Obstetrics and Gynecology* 67 (1986):339-43.

Glover, J. J., D. T. Ozar, and D. C. Thomasma. "Teaching Ethics on Rounds: The Ethicist as Teacher, Consultant, and Decision-Maker." *Theoretical Medicine* 7 (1986):14-31.

Pellegrino, E., R. Hart, and S. Henderson. "Relevance and Utility of Courses in Medical Ethics: A Survey of Physicians' Perceptions." *Journal of the American Medical Association* 253 (1985):49-53.

Pellegrino, E. D., and T. K. McElhinney. *Teaching Ethics, the Humanities, and Human Values in Medical Schools: A Ten Year Overview*. Washington, DC: Institute on Human Values in Medicine, Society for Health and Human Values, 1982.

Perkoff, Gerald T. "Teaching Clinical Medicine in the Ambulatory Setting: An Idea Whose Time May Have Finally Come." *New England Journal of Medicine* 314 (1986):27:31.

Purtilo, Ruth B. "Ethics Teaching in Allied Health Fields." *Hastings Center Report* 8 (April 1978): 14-16.

Rostain, Anthony L., and Marian C. Parrott. "Ethics Committee Simulations for Teaching Medical Ethics." *Journal of Medical Education* 61 (March 1986):178-81.

Siegler, Mark. "A Legacy of Osler: Teaching Clinical Ethics at the Bedside." *Journal of the American Medical Association* 239 (1978):951-56.

Steinfels, M. "Ethics, Education, and Nursing Practice," *Hastings Center Report* 7 (August 1977):20-21.

Part One: Making Treatment Decisions

Cases 1 and 2

Appelbaum, Paul S., and Loren H. Roth. "Clinical Issues in the Assessment of Competency." *American Journal of Psychiatry* 138 (1981):1462-67.

Areen, Judith. "The Legal Status of Consent Obtained from Families of Adult Patients to Withhold or Withdraw Treatment." *Journal of the American Medical Association* 258 (July 10, 1987):229-35.

Cassell, Eric J. "Autonomy in the Intensive Care Unit: The Refusal of Treatment." In *Critical Care Clinics: Ethical Moments in Critical Care Medicine*, II, ed. James P. Orlowski and George Kanote. Philadelphia: W.B. Saunders, 1986.

Childress, James F. *Who Should Decide? Paternalism in Health Care*. New York: Oxford University Press, 1983.

Cohen, Cynthia B. "Ethical Problems of Intensive Care." *Anesthesiology* 47 (1977): 217-27.

Katz, Jay, *The Silent World of Doctor and Patient*. New York: Free Press, 1983.

Kleinig, John. *Paternalism*. Totowa, NJ: Rowman and Allanheld, 1984.

Miller, Bruce L. "Autonomy and the Refusal of Lifesaving Treatment." *Hastings Center Report* 11 (August 1981):22-28.

President's Commission for the Study of Ethical Problems in Medicine and Biomedical and Behavioral Research. *Deciding to Forego Life-Sustaining Treatment*. Washington, DC: U.S. Government Printing Office, 1983.

Roth, Loren H., *et al*. "Tests of Competency to Consent to Treatment." *American Journal of Psychiatry* 134 (1977):279-85.

Ruark, John Edward, Thomas Alfred Raffin, and the Stanford University Medical Center Committee on Ethics. "Initiating and Withdrawing Life Support: Principles and Practice in Adult Medicine." *New England Journal of Medicine* 318 (1988):25-30.

Shultz, Marjorie Maguire. "From Informed Consent to Patient Choice: A New Protected Interest." *Yale Law Journal* 95 (1985):219-99.

Swartz, Martha. "The Patient Who Refuses Medical Treatment: A Dilemma for Hospitals and Physicians." *American Journal of Law and Medicine* 11 (1985):147-94.

Walton, Douglas N. *The Ethics of Withdrawal of Life-Supporting Systems: Case Studies on Decision-Making in Intensive Care*. Westport, CT: Greenwood Press, 1983.

Walton, Douglas N. *Physician-Patient Dcision-Making: A Study in Medical Ethics*. Westport, CT: Greenwood Press, 1985.

Wikler, Daniel. "Paternalism and the Mildly Retarded." *Philosophy and Public Affairs* 8 (Summer 1979):377-92.

Legal Case Cited in Case 1

Bartling v. Superior Court, 163 Cal. App. 3d 186, 209 Cal. Rptr. 220 (Ct. App. 1984), *later appeal, Bartling v. Glendale Adventist Medical Center*, 184 Cal. App. 3d 97, 228 Cal. Rptr. 847 (Ct. App.), *later appeal* 184 Cal. App. 3d 961, 229 Cal. Rptr. 360 (Ct. App. 1986).

Selected Legal Cases on Making Treatment Decisions

In re Conroy, 98 N.J. 321, 486 A.2d 1209 (1985).

In re Eichner (In re Storar), 52 N.Y.2d 363, 420 N.E.2d 64, 438 N.Y.S.2d 266, *cert. denied*, 454 U.S. 858 (1981).

In re Ingram, 102 Wash. 2d 827, 689 P.2d 1363 (1984).

In re Quinlan, 70 N.J. 10, 355 A.2d 647, *cert. denied sub nom. Garger v. New Jersey*, 429 U.S. 922 (1976).

Rennie v. Klein, 462 F. Supp. 1131 (D.N.J.1978).

Satz v. Perlmutter, 362 So. 2d 160 (Fla. Dist. Ct. App. 1978), *aff'd*, 379 So. 2d 359 (Fla. 1980).

In re Schiller, 148 N.J. Super. 168, 372 A.2d 360 (1977).

State Department of Human Services v. Northern, 563 S.W.2d 197, (Tenn. 1978).

Superintendent of Belchertown State School v. Saikewicz, 373 Mass. 728, 370 N.E.2d 417 (1977).

Part Two: Specific Treatment Modalities

A. LONG-TERM LIFE-SUPPORTING TECHNOLOGY

1. Ventilators: Cases 3 and 4

Bosk, Charles L. *Forgive and Remember: Managing Medical Failure.* Chicago: University of Chicago Press, 1979.
Cassem, Ned H. "When to Disconnect the Respirator." *Psychiatric Annals* 9 (1979):38-53.
Devine, Philip E. *The Ethics of Homicide.* Ithaca: Cornell University Press, 1978.
Grenvik, Ake. " 'Terminal Weaning': Discontinuance of Life-Support Therapy in the Terminally Ill Patient." *Critical Care Medicine* 11 (1983):394-95.
Hart, H. L. A., and A. M. Honore. *Causation in the Law.* Oxford: Clarendon Press, 1967.
Horan, Dennis and David Mall. *Death, Dying and Euthanasia.* Washington, DC: University Publications of America, 1977.
Law Reform Commission of Canada. Report 20: *Euthanasia, Aiding Suicide, and Cessation of Treatment.* Ottawa, Canada: November 1983.
Pearlman, Robert A., and Albert Jonsen. "The Use of Quality-of-Life Considerations in Medical Decision Making." *Journal of the American Geriatrics Society* 33 (1985): 344-52.
Winkenwerder, W. "Ethical Dilemmas for House Staff Physicians: The Care of Critically Ill and Dying Patients." *Journal of the American Medical Association* 254 (1985):3454-57.

Selected Legal Cases on Withholding or Withdrawing Ventilators

Barber v. Superior Court, 147 Cal. App. 3d 1006, 195 Cal. Rptr. 484 (Ct. App. 1983).
Bartling v. Superior Court, 163 Cal. App. 3d 186, 209 Cal. Rptr. 220 (Ct. App. 1984), *later appeal, Bartling v. Glendale Adventist Medical Center*, 184 Cal. App. 3d 97, 228 Cal. Rptr. 847 (Ct. App.), *later appeal*, 184 Cal. App. 3d 961, 229 Cal. Rptr. 360 (Ct. App 1986).
In re Colyer, 99 Wash. 2d 114, 660 P.2d 738 (1983).
In re Eichner (In re Storar), 52 N.Y.2d 363, 420 N.E.2d 64, 438 N.Y.S.2d 266, *cert. denied*, 454 U.S. 858 (1981).
In re Farrell, 108 N.J. 335, 529 A.2d 404 (1987).
Foody v. Manchester Memorial Hospital, 40 Conn. Supp. 127, 482 A.2d 713 (Super. Ct. 1984).
In re Hamlin, 689 P.2d 1372 (Wash. 1984).
John F. Kennedy Memorial Hospital, Inc. v. Bludworth, 452 So. 2d 921 (Fla. 1984).
Leach v. Shapiro, 13 Ohio App. 3d 393, 469 N.E.2d 1047 (Ct. App. 1984).
In re Quinlan, 70 N.J. 10, 355 A.2d 647, *cert. denied sub nom., Garger v. New Jersey*, 429 U.S. 922 (1976).
In re Severns, 425 A.2d 156 (Del. Ch. 1980).
In re Torres, 357 N.W. 2d 332 (Minn. 1984).
Satz v. Perlmutter, 362 So. 2d 160 (Fla. Dist. Ct. App. 1978), *aff'd*, 379 So. 2d 359 (Fla. 1980).
Tune v. Walter Reed Army Medical Hospital, 602 F. Supp. 1452 (D.D.C. 1985).

2. Dialysis: Cases 5 and 6

Campbell, James D., and Anne R. Campbell. "The Social and Economic Costs of End-Stage Renal Disease: A Patient's Perspective." *New England Journal of Medicine* 299 (1978):386-92.
Cohen, Cynthia B. " 'Quality of life' and the Analogy with the Nazis." *Journal of Medicine and Philosophy* 8 (1983):113-35.
Evans, Roger W., et al. "The Quality of Life of Patients with End-Stage Renal Disease." *New England Journal of Medicine* 312 (1985): 553-59.
Fox, Renee, C. and Judith P. Swazey, eds. *The Courage to Fail: A Social View of Organ Transplants and Dialysis.* Chicago: University of Chicago Press, 1974.
Katz, Jay, and Alexander M. Capron. *Catastrophic Diseases: Who Decides What? A Psychological and Legal Analysis of the Problems Posed by Hemodialysis and Organ Transplantation.* New York: Russell Sage Foundation, 1975.
Keyserlingk, Edward W. *Sanctity of Life or Quality of Life in the Context of Ethics, Medicine, and Law.* Ottawa: Law Reform Commission of Canada, 1979.
Kilner, J. F. "Selecting Patients When Resources Are Limited: A Study of U.S. Renal Directors." *American Journal of Public Health* [in press].
McCormick, Richard. "The Quality of Life, the Sanctity of Life." *Hastings Center Report* (February 1978):30-36.
Neu, Steven, and Carl M. Kjellstrand. "Stopping Long-Term Dialysis: An Empirical Study of Withdrawal of Life-Supporting Treatment." *New England Journal of Medicine* 314 (January 1986):14-20.
Steinbrook, Robert, et al. "Preferences of Homosexual Men with AIDS for Life-Sustaining Treatment." *New England Journal of Medicine* 314 (1986):457-60.
Thomasma, David C. "Ethical Judgments of Quality of Life in the Care of the Aged." *Journal of the American Geriatrics Society* 32 (1984):525-27.
Westlie, L., et al. "Mortality, Morbidity, and Life Satisfaction in the Very Old Dialysis Patient." *Transactions of the American Society of Artificial Internal Organs* 30 (1984): 21-30.

Selected Legal Cases on Withdrawing or Withholding Dialysis:

In re Lydia E. Hall Hospital, 116 Misc. 2d 477, 455 N.Y.S.2d 706 (Sup. Ct. Nassau County 1982).
New Mexico ex rel. Smith v. Fort, No. 14,768 (N.M. 1983).
In re Spring, 380 Mass. 629, 405 N.E.2d 115 (1980).

B. EMERGENCY INTERVENTIONS

1. Cardiopulmonary Resuscitation: Cases 7 and 8

Bedell, Susanna E., and Thomas L. Delbanco. "Choices about Cardiopulmonary Resuscitation in the Hospital: When Do Physicians Talk with Patients?" *New England Journal of Medicine* 310 (1984):1089-93.
Bedell, Susanna, et al. "Do-Not-Resuscitate Orders for Critically Ill Patients in the Hospital: How Are They Used and What is Their Impact?" *Journal of the American Medical Association* 256 (1986):233-37.
Brennan, Troyen A. "Do-Not-Resuscitate Orders for the Incompetent Patient in the Absence of Family Consent." *Law, Medicine, and Health Care* 14 (1986):13-19.
Charlson, M. E., et al. "Resuscitation: How Do We Decide? A Prospective Study of Physicians' Preferences and the Clinical Course of Hospitalized Patients." *Journal of the American Medical Association* 255 (1986):1316-22.

Evans, Andrew L., and Baruch A. Brody. "The Do-Not-Resuscitate Order in Teaching Hospitals." *Journal of the American Medical Association* 253 (1985):2236-39.

Farber, Neal J., et al. "Cardiopulmonary Resuscitation (CPR): Patient Factors and Decision Making." *Archives of Internal Medicine* 144 (1984):2229-32.

Kellmer, D. M. "No Code Orders: Guidelines for Policy." *Nursing Outlook* 34 (1986):179-83.

Lee, Melinda A., and Christine K. Cassell. "The Ethical and Legal Framework for the Decision Not to Resuscitate." *Western Journal of Medicine* 140 (1984):117-22.

Lewandowski, Wendy, et al. "Treatment and Care of 'Do Not Resuscitate' Patients in a Medical Intensive Care Unit." *Heart and Lung* 14 (1985):175-81.

Lipton, Helene L. "Do-Not-Resuscitate Decisions in a Community Hospital." *Journal of the American Medical Association* 256 (1986):1164-69.

Lo, Bernard, et al. "Do Not Resuscitate Decisions: A Prospective Study of Three Teaching Hospitals." *Archives of Internal Medicine* 145 (1985):1115-17.

Lo, Bernard, and Robert L. Steinbrook. "Deciding Whether to Resuscitate." *Archives of Internal Medicine* 143 (1983):1561-63.

Miles, Steven H., and D. C. Moldow. "The Prevalence and Design of Hospital Protocols Limiting Medical Treatment." *Archives of Internal Medicine* 144 (1984): 1841-43.

Miles, Steven H., and Timothy J. Crimmins. "Orders to Limit Emergency Treatment for an Ambulance Service in a Large Metropolitan Area." *Journal of the American Medical Association* 254 (1985):525-27.

National Conference on Cardiopulmonary Resuscitation (CPR) and Emergency Cardiac Care (ECC). "Standards and Guidelines for Cardiopulmonary Resuscitation (CPR) and Emergency Cardiac Care (ECC)." *Journal of the American Medical Association* 255 (1986):2905-84.

Nolan, Kathleen. "In Death's Shadow: The Meanings of Withholding Resuscitation." *Hastings Center Report* 17 (October–November 1987):9-14.

Schwartz, D. A., and P. Reilly. "The Choice Not to Be Resuscitated." *Journal of the American Geriatric Society* 34 (1986):807-11.

Stephens, R. L. " 'Do not Resuscitate' Orders: Ensuring the Patient's Participation." *Journal of the American Medical Association* 255 (1986):240-41.

Tomlinson, Tom, and Howard Brody. "Ethics and Communication in Do-Not-Resuscitate Orders." *New England Journal of Medicine* 318 (1988):43-46.

Veatch, Robert M. "Deciding against Resuscitation: Encouraging Signs and Potential Dangers." *Journal of the American Medical Association* 253 (1985):77-78.

Youngner, Stuart J. "Do Not Resuscitate Orders: No Longer Secret, but Still a Problem." *Hastings Center Report* 17 (February 1987):24-33.

Zimmerman, J. E., et al. "The Use and Implications of Do-Not-Resuscitate Orders in Intensive Care Units." *Journal of the American Medical Association* 255 (1986): 351-56.

Selected Legal Cases on Do Not Resuscitate Orders

Brophy v. New England Sinai Hospital, 398 Mass. 417, 497 N.E.2d 626 (1986).
In re Dinnerstein, 6 Mass. App. 466, 380 N.E.2d 134 (App. Ct. 1978).
In re Hamlin, 689 P.2d 1372 (Wash. 1984).

2. Life-Threatening Bleeding: Cases 9 and 10

Besdine, Richard W. "Decisions to Withhold Treatment from Nursing Home Residents." *Journal of the American Geriatrics Society* 31 (1983):602-6.

Crosby, L. A. "Not on My Shift." *Journal of the American Medical Association* 253 (1985):1402.

Dixon, J. Lowell, and M. Gene Smalley. "Jehovah's Witnesses: The Surgical/Ethical Challenge." *Journal of the American Medical Association* 246 (1981):2471-72.

Drew, N. C. "The Pregnant Jehovah's Witness." *Journal of Medical Ethics* 7 (1981):137-39.

Findley, Larry J., and Paul M. Redstone. "Blood Transfusion in Adult Jehovah's Witnesses: A Case Study of One Congregation." *Archives of Internal Medicine* (1982): 606-7.

Jonsen, Albert R. "Blood Transfusions and Jehovah's Witnesses: The Impact of the Patient's Unusual Beliefs in Critical Care." *Critical Care Clinics* 2 (1986):91-100.

Lynn, Joanne D. "Ethical Issues in Caring for Elderly Residents of Nursing Homes." *Primary Care* 13 (1986):295-306.

Macklin, Ruth. "Consent, Coercion and Conflicts of Rights." *Perspectives in Biology and Medicine* (Spring 1977):360-71.

Medical Department, World Headquarters of Jehovah's Witnesses. "Professionally Speaking: Refusal of Blood—An Ethical Issue?" *Journal of the American Medical Association* 246 (1981):2471-72.

Swartz, Martha. "The Patient Who Refuses Medical Treatment: A Dilemma for Hospitals and Physicians." *American Journal of Law and Medicine* 11 (1985):147-94.

Selected Legal Cases on Withholding or Withdrawing Treatment for Life-Threatening Bleeding

In re Estate of Brooks, 32 Ill. 2d 361, 205 N.E. 2d 435 (1965).

Commissioner of Corrections v. Myers, 399 N.E.2d 452 (Mass. 1979).

Erickson v. Dilgard, 44 Misc. 2d 27, 252 N.Y.S.2d 705 (1962).

Application of President and Directors of Georgetown College, 331 F.2d 1000 (D.C. Cir), *cert. denied*, 377 U.S. 978 (1964).

Hamilton v. McAuliffe, 277 Md. 336, 353 A.2d 634 (1976).

Holmes v. Silver Cross Hospital, 340 F. Supp. 125 (N.D. Ill. 1972).

John F. Kennedy Memorial Hospital v. Heston, 58 N.J. 576, 279 A.2d 670 (1971).

In re Melideo 88 Misc 2d 974, 390 N.Y.S. 2d 523 (1976).

In re Osborne, 294 A. 2d 372 (D.C. 1972).

Raleigh Fitkin-Paul Morgan Memorial Hospital v. Anderson, 42 N.J. 421, 201 A.2d 537, *cert. denied* 377 U.S. 985 (1964).

In re Storar, 52 N.Y.2d 363, 420 N.E.2d 64, 438 N.Y.S.2d 266, *cert. denied*, 454 U.S. 858 (1981).

United States v. George, 239 F. Supp. 752 (D. Conn. 1965).

C. MEDICAL PROCEDURES FOR SUPPLYING NUTRITION AND HYDRATION

Cases 11 and 12

American Medical Association, Council on Ethical and Judicial Affairs. "Statement on Withholding or Withdrawing Life Prolonging Treatment." March 15, 1986.

Annas, George J. "Fashion and Freedom: When Artificial Feeding Should Be Withdrawn." *American Journal of Public Health* 75 (1985):685-88.

———"Do Feeding Tubes Have More Rights than Patients?" *Hastings Center Report* 16 (February 1986):26-28.

Barry, Robert. "Facing Hard Cases: The Ethics of Assisted Feeding." *Issues in Law and Medicine* 2 (September 1986):99-115.

Benjamin, Martin, and Joy Curtis. "Ethical Autonomy in Nursing." In *Health Care Ethics*, ed. Donald VanDeVeer and Tom Regan. Philadelphia: Temple University Press, 1987.

Billings, J. A. "Comfort Measures for the Terminally Ill: Is Dehydration Painful?" *Journal of the American Geriatrics Society* 33 (1985):808-10.

Callahan, Daniel. "On Feeding the Dying." *Hastings Center Report* 13 (October 1983):22.

Capron, Alexander M. "Ironies and Tensions in Feeding the Dying." *Hastings Center Report* 14 (October 1984):32-35.

Chang, R. W. S., S. Jacobs, and B. Lee. "Use of Apache II Severity of Disease Classification to Identify Intensive-Care-Unit Patients Who Would Not Benefit from Total Parenteral Nutrition." *Lancet* 1, no. 8496 (June 28, 1986):1483-87.

Connery, John R. "The Ethical Standards for Withholding/Withdrawing Nutrition and Hydration." *Issues in Law and Medicine* 2 (September 1986):87-97.

Curran, William J. "Defining Appropriate Medical Care: Providing Nutrients and Hydration for the Dying." *New England Journal of Medicine* 313 (1985):940-42.

Derr, Patrick. "Why Food and Fluids Can Never Be Denied." *Hastings Center Report* 16 (February 1986):28-30.

Dresser, R. S., and E. V. Boisaubin, "Ethics, Law, and Nutritional Support." *Archives of Internal Medicine* 145 (1985):122-24.

Green, Willard. "Setting Boundaries for Artificial Feeding." *Hastings Center Report* 14 (December 1984):8-11.

Horan, D. J. and E. R. Grant. "The Legal Aspects of Withholding Nourishment." *Journal of Legal Medicine* 5, no. 11984:595-632.

King, Dorothy G., and Julie O'Sullivan Maillet. Position of the American Dietetic Association: "Issues in Feeding the Terminally Ill Adult." *Journal of the American Dietetic Association* (January 1987):78-85.

Lo, Bernard, and Laurie Dornbrand. "Sounding Board: Guiding the Hand that Feeds: Caring for the Demented Elderly." *New England Journal of Medicine* 311 (1984): 402-4.

Lyn gh, Joan. "Narrow Passageways: Nurses and Physicians in Conflict and Concert since 1875." In *The Physician as Captain of the Ship: A Critical Reappraisal*, eds. Tristam Englehardt and Stuart Spicker. Boston: D. Reidel, 1987.

Lynn, Joanne D. "Ethical Issues in Caring for Elderly Residents of Nursing Homes." *Primary Care* 13 (1986):295-306.

Lynn, Joanne, ed. *By No Extraordinary Means: The Choice to Forgo Life-Sustaining Food and Water*. Bloomington: Indiana University Press, 1986.

Lynn, Joanne, and James F. Childress. "Must Patients Always Be Given Food and Water?" *Hastings Center Report* 13 (October 1983):17-21.

Meilander, Gilbert. "On Removing Food and Water: Against the Stream." *Hastings Center Report* 14 (December 1984): 11-13.

Meyers, D. W. "Legal Aspects of Withdrawing Nourishment from an Incurably Ill Patient." *Archives of Internal Medicine* 145 (1985):125-28.

Micetich, K. C., P. H. Steinecker, and D. C. Thomasma. "Are Intravenous Fluids Morally Required for a Dying Patient?" *Archives of Internal Medicine* 143 (1983):975-78.

Miles, Steven. "The Terminally Ill Elderly: Dealing with the Ethics of Feeding," *Geriatrics* 40 (1985):112-20.

Mitchell, Christine. "Integrity in Interprofessional Relationships." In *Responsibility in Health Care*, ed. George J. Agich. Dordrecht, Holland: D. Reidel, 1981.

O'Rourke, Kevin. "The A.M.A. Statement on Tube Feeding: An Ethical Analysis." *America* 155 (1986):321-23, 331.

Paris, John J. "When Burdens of Feeding Outweigh Benefits," *Hastings Center Report* (February 1986):30-32.

Paris, John J., and Anne Fletcher. "Infant Doe Regulations and the Absolute Requirement to Use Nourishment and Fluids for the Dying Patient." *Law, Medicine, and Health Care* 11 (1983):210-13.

Siegler, Mark, and Alan J. Weisbard. "Against the Emerging Stream: Should Fluids and Nutritional Support Be Discontinued?" *Archives of Internal Medicine* 145 (January 1985): 129-31.

Wanzer, Sidney, *et al.*. "The Physician's Responsibility Toward Hopelessly Ill Patients." *New England Journal of Medicine* 310 (1984):955-59.

Watts, D. T., and Christine K. Cassel. "Extraordinary Nutritional Support: A Case Study and Ethical Analysis." *Journal of the American Geriatrics Society* 32 (1984): 237-42.

Watts, D. T., Christine K. Cassel, and D. H. Hickam. "Nurses' and Physicians' Attitudes toward Tube-Feeding Decisions in Long-Term Care." *Journal of the American Geriatrics Society* 34 (1986):607-11.

Winslow, Gerald R. "From Loyalty to Advocacy: A New Metaphor for Nursing." *Hastings Center Report* 14 (June 1984):32-40.

Zerwekh, Joyce V. "The Dehydration Question." *Nursing 83* (1983):47-51.

Selected Legal Cases on Withdrawing or Withholding
Artificial Nutrition and Hydration

Barber v. Superior Court, 147 Cal. App. 3d 1006, 195 Cal. Rptr. 484 (Ct. App. 1983).

Bouvia v. Superior Court (Glenchur), 179 Cal. App. 3d 1127, 225 Cal. Rptr. 297 (Ct. App.), *review denied* (Cal. June 5, 1986).

Brophy v. New England Sinai Hospital, Inc., 398 Mass. 417, 497 N.E.2d 626 (1986).

In re Conroy, 98 N.J. 321, 486 A.2d 1209 (1985).

Corbett v. D'Alessandro, 487 So. 2d 368 (Fla. Dist. Ct. App.), *review denied,* 492 So. 2d 1331 (Fla. 1986).

In re Hier, 18 Mass. App. Ct. 200, 464 N.E. 2d 959, *review denied,* 392 Mass. 1102, 465 N.E. 2d 261 (1984).

In re Jobes, 108 N.J. 394, 529 A.2d 434 (1987).

In re Peter, 108 N.J. 365, 529 A.2d 419 (1987).

In re Requena, 213 N.J. Super. 475, 517 A.2d 886 (Super. Ct. Ch. Div.), *aff'd.* 213 N.J. Super. 443, 517 A.2d 869 (Super. Ct. App. Div. 1986) (per curiam).

In re Rodas, (Colo. Dist. Ct. Mesa County Jan. 22, 1987)

In re Severns, 425 A. 2d 156 (Del. Ch. 1980).

D. ANTIBIOTICS AND OTHER LIFE-SUSTAINING MEDICATION

Cases 13 and 14

Besdine, Richard W. "Decisions to Withhold Treatment from Nursing Home Residents." *Journal of the American Geriatrics Society* 31 (1983):602-6.

Boyle, Joseph. "On Killing and Letting Die." *New Scholasticism* 51 (1977):433-52.

Braithwaite, Susan, and David C. Thomasma. "New Guidelines on Foregoing Life-Sustaining Treatment in Incompetent Patients: An Anticruelty Policy." *Annals of Internal Medicine* 104 (1986): 711-15.

Brock, Dan W. "Taking Human Life." *Ethics* 95 (1985):851-65.

Brown, Norman K., and Donovan J. Thompson. "Nontreatment of Fever in Extended Care Facilities." *New England Journal of Medicine* 300 (1979):1246-50.

Clouser, K. Danner. "Allowing or Causing: Another Look." *Annals of Internal Medicine* 87 (1977):622-24.

Cohen, Cynthia B. " 'Quality of Life' and the Analogy with the Nazis." *Journal of Medicine and Philosophy* 8 (1983):113-35.

Foot, Philippa. "Euthanasia." *Philosophy and Public Affairs* 6 (1977):85-112.

Hilfiker, David. "Allowing the Debilitated to Die: Facing Our Ethical Choices." *New England Journal of Medicine* 308 (1983):716-19.

Horan, Dennis, and David Mall. *Death, Dying, and Euthanasia*. Washington, DC: University Publications of America, 1977.

Keyserlingk, Edward W. *Sanctity of Life or Quality of Life in the Context of Ethics, Medicine, and Law*. Ottawa: Law Reform Commission of Canada, 1979.

Kohn, R. R. "Causes of Death in Very Old People." *Journal of the American Medical Association* 247 (1982):2793-97.

Lynn, Joanne D. "Ethical Issues in Caring for Elderly Residents of Nursing Homes." *Primary Care* 13 (1986):295-306.

McCormick, Richard. "The Quality of Life, the Sanctity of Life." *Hastings Center Report* (February 1978):30-36.

Rachels, James. *The End of Life: Euthanasia and Morality*. Oxford: Oxford University Press, 1986.

Thomasma, David C. "Ethical Judgments of Quality of Life in the Care of the Aged." *Journal of the American Geriatrics Society* 32 (1984):525-27.

Wanzer, Sidney, *et al.* "The Physician's Responsibility toward Hopelessly Ill Patients." *New England Journal of Medicine* 310 (1984):955-59.

Zimmer, J. G. *et al.* "Systemic Antibiotic Use in Nursing Homes: A Quality Assessment." *Journal of the American Geriatrics Society* 34 (1986):703-10.

Selected Legal Cases on Withholding or Withdrawing Antibiotics

Brophy v. New England Sinai Hospital, Inc., 398 Mass. 417, 497 N.E.2d 626 (1986).

In re Hamlin, 689 P.2d 1372 (Wash. 1984).

In re Severns, 425 A. 2d 156 (Del. Ch. 1980).

E. PALLIATIVE CARE AND THE RELIEF OF PAIN

Cases 15 and 16

Angell, Marcia. "The Quality of Mercy." *New England Journal of Medicine* 306 (1982):98-99.

Bonica, John. J., and Vittorio Ventafridda, eds. *International Symposium on Pain of Advanced Cancer: Advances in Pain Research Therapy*, II. New York: Raven Press, 1979.

Cassell, Eric J. "The Relief of Suffering." *Archives of Internal Medicine* 143 (1983): 522-23.

Cushing, Maureen. "Cause of Death: Drug or Disease? *American Journal of Nursing* 83 (1983):943-44.

Foley, Kathleen M. "The Treatment of Cancer Pain." *New England Journal of Medicine* 313 (1985):84-95.

Kane, R. L., L. Bernstein, J. Wales, and R. Rothenberg. "Hospice Effectiveness in Controlling Pain." *Journal of the American Medical Association* 253 (1985):2683-86.

Lynn, Joanne. "Care Near the End of Life." In *Geriatric Medicine, II. Fundamentals of Geriatric Care*, ed. Christine K. Cassel and John R. Walsh. New York: Springer Verlag, 1984.

Marks, Richard M., and Edward J. Sachar. "Undertreatment of Medical Inpatients with Narcotic Analgesics." *Annals of Internal Medicine* 78 (1973):173-81.

McCormick, Richard A., and Paul Ramsey, eds. *Doing Evil to Achieve Good: Moral Choice in Conflict Situations*. Chicago: Loyola University Press, 1978.

Melzack, Ronald. *The Challenge of Pain*. New York: Basic Books, 1982.
Porter, Jane, and Hershel Jick. "Addiction Rare in Patients Treated with Narcotics." *New England Journal of Medicine* 302 (1980):123.
Saunders, Cicely M., ed. *The Management of Terminal Disease*. London: Edward Arnold, 1978.
The Task Force on Supportive Care. "The Supportive Care Plan—Its Meaning and Application: Recommendations and Guidelines." *Law, Medicine, and Health Care* 12 (June 1984):97-102.
Vere, D. W. "The Hospital as a Place of Pain." *Journal of Medical Ethics* (1980): 117-19.

Part Three: Prospective Planning: Advance Directives

Cases 17 and 18

"Appointing an Agent to Make Medical Treatment Choices." *Columbia Law Review* 84 (1984):985-1025.
Bosk, Charles L. *Forgive and Remember: Managing Medical Failure*. Chicago: University of Chicago Press, 1979.
Eisendrath, Stuart J., and Albert R. Jonsen. "The Living Will: Help or Hindrance?" *Journal of the American Medical Association* 249 (1983):2054-58.
Miles, Steven H. "Advance Directives to Limit Treatment: The Need for Portability." *Journal of the American Geriatrics Society* 35 (1987):74-76.
Mishkin, Barbara. *A Matter of Choice: Planning Ahead for Health Care Decisions*. Washington, DC: American Association of Retired Persons, 1986.
President's Commission for the Study of Ethical Problems in Medicine and Biomedical and Behavioral Research. *Deciding to Forego Life-Sustaining Treatment: Ethical, Medical, and Legal Issues in Treatment Decisions*. Washington, DC: U.S. Government Printing Office, 1983.
Schneiderman, Lawrence J., and John D. Arras. "Counseling Patients to Counsel Physicians on Future Care in the Event of Patient Incompetence." *Annals of Internal Medicine* 102 (1985):693-98.
Society for the Right to Die. *The Physician and the Hopelessly Ill Patient: Legal, Medical, and Ethical Guidelines*. New York: Society for the Right to Die, 1984.
———*Handbook of Living Will Laws: 1987 Edition*. New York: Society for the Right to Die, 1988.
Steinbrook, R., and B. Lo. "Decisionmaking for Incompetent Patients by Designated Proxy." *New England Journal of Medicine* 310 (1984): 1598-1601.
Winkenwerder, W. "Ethical Dilemmas for House Staff Physicians: The Care of Critically Ill and Dying Patients." *Journal of the American Medical Association* 254 (1985):3454-57.

Selected Legal Cases on Advance Directives

Bartling V. Superior Court, 163 Cal. App. 3d 186, 209 Cal. Rptr. 220 (Ct. App. 1984), *later appeal*, *Bartling v. Glendale Adventist Medical Center*, 184 Cal. App. 3d 97, 228 Cal. Rptr. 847 (Ct. App.), *later appeal*, 184 Cal. App. 3d 961, 229 Cal. Rptr. 360 (Ct. App. 1986).
In re Conroy, 98 N.J. 321, 486 A.2d 1209 (1985).
John F. Kennedy Memorial Hospital v. Bludworth, 452 So. 2d 921 (Fla. 1984).

In re Peter, 108 N.J. 365, 529 A.2d 419 (1987).
Saunders v. State, 129 Misc. 2d 45, 492 N.Y.S.2d 510 (Sup. Ct. 1985).

Part Four: Declaring Death

Cases 19 and 20

Cranford, Ronald E. "Termination of Treatment in the Persistent Vegetative State." *Seminars in Neurology* 4 (March 1984):36-44.
Cranford, Ronald E., and Harmon Smith. "Some Critical Distinctions between Brain Death and the Persistent Vegetative State." *Ethics in Science and Medicine (1979):* 199-209.
Grenvik, Ake, *et al.* "Cessation of Therapy in Terminal Illness and Brain Death." *Critical Care Medicine* 6 (1978)284-91.
Lynn, Joanne. "The Determination of Death." *Annals of Internal Medicine* 99 (1983):264-66.
President's Commission for the Study of Ethical Problems in Medicine and Biomedical and Behavioral Research. *Defining Death: Medical, Legal, and Ethical Issues in the Determination of Death.* Washington, DC: U.S. Government Printing Office, 1981.
Shrader, Douglas. "On Dying More than One Death." *Hastings Center Report* 16 (February 1986):12-16.
Veatch, Robert M. "The Definition of Death: Ethical, Philosophical, and Policy Confusion." *Annals of the New York Academy of Science* 315 (1978):307-21.
————*Death, Dying, and the Biological Revolution.* New Haven: Yale University Press, 1976.
Veith, Frank, *et al.* "Brain Death: I: A Status Report of Medical and Ethical Considerations." "II: A Status Report of Legal Considerations." *Journal of the American Medical Association* 238 (October 10 and 17, 1977):1651-55, 1744-48.
Walton, Douglas N. *On Defining Death: An Analytic Study of the Concept of Death in Philosophy and Medical Ethics.* Montreal: McGill-Queen's University Press, 1979.

Selected Legal Cases Distinguishing Treatment of Patients in
Persistent Vegetative State from Treatment of Patients Declared Dead

Brophy v. New England Sinai Hospital, Inc., 398 Mass. 417, 497 N.E.2d 626 (1986).
In re Colyer, 99 Wash. 2d 114, 660 P.2d 738 (1983).
Corbett v. D'Alessandro, 487 So. 2d 368 (Fla. Dist. Ct. App.), *review denied*, 492 So. 2d 1331 (Fla. 1986).
In re Eichner (In re Storar), 52 N.Y.2d 363, 4209 N.E.2d 64, 438 N.Y.S.2d 266, *cert. denied*, 454 U.S. 858 (1981).
Foody v. Manchester Memorial Hospital, 40 Conn. Supp. 127, 482 A.2d 713 (Super. Ct. 1984).
In re Jobes, 108 N.J. 394, 529 A.2d 434 (1987).
John F. Kennedy Memorial Hospital v. Bludworth, 452 So. 2d 921 (Fla. 1984).
Leach v. Shapiro, 13 Ohio App. 3d 393, 469 N.E.2d 1047 (Ct. App. 1984).
In re Peter, 108 N.J. 365, 529 A.2d 419 (1987).
In re Quinlan, 70 N.J. 10, 355 A.2d 647, *cert denied sub nom.*, *Garger v. New Jersey*, 429 U.S. 922 (1976).
Rasmussen v. Fleming, No. CV-86-0450 PR (Ariz. July 23, 1987).
In re Severns, 425 A. 2d 156 (Del. Ch. 1980).

Part Five: Policy Considerations

A. ETHICS COMMITTEES

Cases 21 and 22

Cohen, Cynthia B. "The Birth of a Network." *Hastings Center Report* 18 (January-February 1988):11-12.

————"Interdisciplinary Consultation on the Care of the Critically Ill and Dying: The Role of One Hospital Ethics Committee." *Critical Care Medicine* 10 (1982):776-84.

Cranford, Ronald E., *et al.* "Institutional Ethics Committees: Issues of Confidentiality and Immunity." *Law, Medicine, and Health Care* 13 (April 1985):52-60.

Cranford, Ronald E., and A. Edward Doudera, eds. *Institutional Ethics Committees and Health Care Decision Making.* Ann Arbor, MI: Health Administration Press, 1984.

Fost, Norman, and Ronald Cranford. "Hospital Ethics Committees: Administrative Aspects." *Journal of the American Medical Association* 253 (1985):2687-92.

Gibson, Joan McIver, and Thomasine Kimbrough Kushner. "Will the 'Conscience of an Institution' Become Society's Servant?" *Hastings Center Report* 16 (June 1986): 9-11.

Hosford, Bowen. *Bioethics Committees.* Rockville, MD: Aspen Systems Corporation, 1986.

Lo, Bernard. "Behind Closed Doors: Promises and Pitfalls of Ethics Committees." *New England Journal of Medicine* 317 (July 2, 1987):46-50.

McCormick, Richard A. "Ethics Committees: Promise or Peril?" *Law, Medicine, and Health Care* 12 (September, 1984):150-55.

Merritt, Andrew L. "Assessing the Risk of Legal Liability of Ethics Committees." *Hastings Center Report* 18 (January-February 1988):13-14.

————"The Tort Liability of Hospital Ethics Committees." *Southern California Law Review* 60 (July, 1987):1239-97.

Murray, Thomas. "Where Are the Ethics in Ethics Committees?" *Hastings Center Report* 18 (January-February 1988):12-13.

President's Commission for the Study of Ethical Problems in Medicine and Biomedical and Behavioral Research. *Deciding to Forego Life-Sustaining Treatment.* Washington, DC: U.S. Government Printing Office, 1983.

Robertson, John A. "Ethics Committees in Hospitals: Alternative Structures and Responsibilities." *Quality Review Bulletin* (January 1984):6-10.

Rosner, Fred. "Hospital Medical Ethics Committees: A Review of Their Development." *Journal of the American Medical Association* 253 (1985):2693-97.

Ross, Judith Wilson. *Handbook for Hospital Ethics Committees.* American Hospital Association Publishing, 1986.

Siegler, Mark. "Ethics Committees: Decisions by Bureaucracy." *Hastings Center Report* 16 (June 1986):22-24.

Wolf, Susan M. "Ethics Committees in the Courts." *Hastings Center Report* 16 (June 1986):12-15.

Selected Legal Cases on Institutional Ethics Committees

Bouvia v. Glenchur, No. C583828 (L.A. Super. Ct. filed Oct. 7, 1986).

In re Eichner (In re Storar), 52 N.Y.2d 363, 420 N.E.2d 64, 438 N.Y.S.2d 266, *cert. denied*, 454 U.S. 858 (1981).

John F. Kennedy Memorial Hospital v. Bludworth, 452 So. 2d 921 (Fla. 1984).
In re Quinlan, 70 N.J. 10, 355 A.2d 647, *cert. denied sub nom. Garger v. New Jersey*, 429 U.S. 922 (1976).
In re Torres, 357 N.W.2d 332 (Minn. 1984).
Superintendent of Belchertown State School v. Saikewicz, 373 Mass. 629, 405 N.E.2d 115 (Mass. 1977).

B. INSTITUTIONAL POLICIES FOR PATIENT ADMISSIONS AND TRANSFERS

Cases 23 and 24

American College of Emergency Physicians. "Guidelines for Transfer of Patients." *Annals of Emergency Medicine* 14 (1985):1221-22.
Besdine, R. W. "Decisions to Withhold Treatment from Nursing Home Residents." *Journal of the American Geriatrics Society* 31 (1983):602-6.
Braunstein, C., and R. Schlenker. "The Impact of Change in Medicare Payment for Acute Care." *Geriatric Nursing* 6 (1985):266-70.
Cohen, Cynthia B. "Ethical Problems of Intensive Care." *Anesthesiology* 47 (1977): 217-27.
Davis, Karen, and Diane Rawland. "Uninsured and Underserved: Inequities in Health Care in the U.S." In President's Commission for the Study of Ethical Problems in Medicine and Biomedical and Behavioral Research, *Securing Access to Health Care: The Ethical Implications of Differences in the Availability of Health Services*. Vol. III. Appendices: Empirical, Legal, and Conceptual Studies. Washington, DC: U.S. Government Printing Office, 1983.
Englehardt, Jr., H. Tristam, and Michael A. Rie. "Intensive Care Units, Scarce Resources, and Conflicting Principles of Justice." *Journal of the American Medical Association* 255 (1986):1159-64.
Gardner, Karen, ed. *Quality of Care for the Terminally Ill: An Examination of the Issues*. Chicago: Joint Commission on Accreditation of Hospitals, 1985.
Gillick, Muriel, and K. Steel. "Referral of Patients from Long-Term Care: An Examination of Transfers." *Journal of the American Geriatrics Society* 31 (1983):74-78.
Himmelstein, D. U., *et al.* "Patient Transfers: Medical Practice As Social Triage." *American Journal of Public Health* 74 (1984):494-97.
Horn, Susan Dadakis. "Measuring Severity of Illness: Comparisons Across Institutions." *American Journal of Public Health* 73 (1983):25-31.
Iglehart, John. "Medical Care of the Poor—A Growing Problem." *New England Journal of Medicine* 313 (1985):59-63.
Irvine, P., N. Van Buren, and K. Crossley. "Causes for Hospitalization of Nursing Home Residents." *Journal of the American Geriatrics Society* 32 (1984):103-7.
Knaus, W. A., *et al.* "An Evaluation of Outcomes from Intensive Care in Major Medical Centers." *Annals of Internal Medicine* 104 (1986):410-18.
Koren, M. J. "Home Care—Who Cares?" *New England Journal of Medicine* 314 (1986):917-20.
Lind, Stuart E. "Transferring the Terminally Ill." *New England Journal of Medicine* 311 (1984):1181-82.
Lynn, Joanne. "Ethics in Hospice Care." In *Hospice Handbook: A Guide for Managers*, ed. Lenora Finn Paradis. Rockville, MD: Aspen Systems, 1985.
Miles, S. H., and M. D. Ryden. "Limited Treatment Policies in Long-Term Care Facilities." *Journal of the American Geriatrics Society* 33 (1985):707-11.
Murphy, Catherine. "The Changing Role of Nurses in Making Ethical Decisions." *Law, Medicine, and Health Care* (September 1984):173-75, 184.

Perkins, Henry S., *et al*. "Providers as Predictors: Using Outcome Predictions in Intensive care." *Critical Care Medicine* 14 (1986):105-10.

Reed, William G., Karen A. Cawley, and Ron J. Anderson. "The Effect of a Public Hospital's Transfer Policy on Patient Care." *New England Journal of Medicine* 315 (1986):1428-32.

Relman, Arnold S. "Texas Eliminates Dumping: A Start toward Equity in Hospital Care." *New England Journal of Medicine* 314 (1986):578-79.

Schiff, Robert L., *et al*. "Transfers to a Public Hospital: A Prospective Study of 467 Patients." *New England Journal of Medicine* 314 (1986):552-57.

Starr, Paul. *The Social Transformation of American Medicine*. New York: Basic Books, 1982.

Tresch, D. D., W. M. Simpson, and J. R. Burton. "Relationship of Long-Term and Acute Care Facilities: The Problem of Patient Transfer and Continuity of Care." *Journal of the American Geriatrics Society* 33 (1985):819-26.

Zawacki, Bruce E. "ICU Physician's Ethical Role in Distributing Scarce Resources." *Critical Care Medicine* 13 (1985):57-60.

Selected Legal Case on Transfers

Bouvia v. County of Riverside, No. 159780 (Super Ct. Calif. Dec. 16, 1983).

In re Peter, 108 N.J. 365, 529 A.2d 419 (1987).

In re Requena, 213 N.J. Super. 475, 517 A.2d 886 (Super Ct. Ch. Div.), aff'd. 213 N.J. Super. 443, 517 A.2d 869 (Super Ct. App. Div. 1986) (per curiam).

Thompson v. Sun City Community Hospital, No. 16634-Pr, slip. op. (Ariz. July 12, 1984).

C. THE USE OF ECONOMIC CONSIDERATIONS IN DECISIONS
CONCERNING LIFE-SUSTAINING TREATMENTS

Cases 25 and 26

Aaron, Henry J., and William B. Schwartz. *The Painful Prescription: Rationing Hospital Care*. Washington, DC: The Brookings Institution, 1984.

Angell, Marcia. "Cost Containment and the Physician." *Journal of the American Medical Association* 254 (September 1985):1203-7.

Avorn, Jerome L. "Benefit and Cost Analysis in Geriatric Care, Turning Age Discrimination into Health Policy." *New England Journal of Medicine* 310 (1984):1294-1301.

Bayer, Ronald, *et al*. "The Care of the Terminally Ill: Morality and Economics." *New England Journal of Medicine* 309 (December 1983):1490-94.

Bayles, Michael D. "The Price of Life." *Ethics* 89 (1978):20-32.

Boyle, Joseph F. "Should We Learn to Say No?" *Journal of the American Medical Association* 252 (1984):782-84.

Brock, Dan W., and Allen Buchanan. "Ethical Issues in For-Profit Health Care." In *For-Profit Enterprise in Health Care*, ed. Bradford H. Gray. Washington, DC: National Academy Press, 1986.

Buchanan, Allen. "Justice: A Philosophical Review." In *Justice and Health Care*, ed. Earl Shelp. Dordrecht, Holland: D. Reidel, 1981.

Bunker, John P. "When Doctors Disagree." *The New York Review of Books* (April 25, 1985):7-12.

Daniels, Norman. "Why Saying No to Patients in the United States Is So Hard: Cost Containment, Justice, and Provider Autonomy." *New England Journal of Medicine* 314 (May 1986):1380-83.

Eisenberg, John M. *Doctors' Decisions and the Cost of Medical Care*. Ann Arbor, MI:Health Administration Press, 1986.

Evans, Roger W. "Health Care Technology and the Inevitability of Resource Allocation and Rationing Decisions." Parts I and II. *Journal of the American Medical Association* 249 (1983):2047-53, 2208-19.

Fein, Rashi. *Medical Care, Medical Costs: The Search for a Health Insurance Policy*. Cambridge: Harvard University Press, 1986.

Fuchs, Victor. *The Health Economy*. Cambridge: Harvard University Press, 1986.

Ginzberg, Eli. "The Monetarization of Medical Care." *New England Journal of Medicine* 310 (1984):1162-65.

Iglehart, John. "Medical Care of the Poor—A Growing Problem." *New England Journal of Medicine* 313 (1985):59-63.

Johnson, Dana E. "Life, Death, and the Dollar Sign: Medical Ethics and Cost Containment." *Journal of the American Medical Association* 252 (1984):223-24.

Lave, Judith R., and William A. Knaus. "The Economics of Intensive Care Units." In *Medicolegal Aspects of Critical Care*, ed. K. Benesch, *et al.* Rockville, MD: Aspen Publishers, 1986.

Leaf, Alexander. "The Doctor's Dilemma—And Society's Too." *New England Journal of Medicine* 310 (1984):718-20.

Mechanic, David. *From Advocacy to Allocation: The Evolving American Health Care System*. New York: The Free Press, 1986.

Menzel, Paul T. *Medical Costs, Moral Choices: A Philosophy of Health Care Economics in America*. New Haven: Yale University Press, 1983.

Mundinger, Mary O'Neil. "Health Service Funding Cuts and the Declining Health of the Poor." *New England Journal of Medicine* 313 (1985):44-47.

Pellegrino, Edmund D. "Rationing Health Care: The Ethics of Medical Gatekeeping." *Journal of Contemporary Health, Law, and Policy* 2 (1986)23-45.

President's Commission for the Study of Ethical Problems in Medicine and Biomedical and Behavioral Research. *Securing Access to Health Care: The Ethical Implications of Differences in the Availability of Health Services*, I. Washington, DC: U.S. Government Printing Office, 1983.

Relman, Arnold S. "Economic Considerations in Emergency Care: What Are Hospitals For?" *New England Journal of Medicine* 312 (1985):372-73.

Schramm, Carl J. "Can We Solve the Hospital-Cost Problem in Our Democracy? *New England Journal of Medicine* 311 (1984):729-32.

Schroeder, Steven A. "Doctors and the Medical Cost Crisis: Culprits, Victims or Solution?" *The Pharos* 48 (Spring, 1985):12-18.

Schwartz, William B. "The Inevitable Failure of Current Cost-Containment Strategies:Why They Can Provide Only Temporary Relief. *Journal of the American Medical Association* 257 (1987):220-24.

Scitovsky, Ann A., and Alexander M. Capron. "Medical Care at the End of Life: The Interaction of Economics and Ethics." *Annual Review of Public Health* 7 (1986):71.

Showstack, Jonathan A., *et al.* "The Role of Changing Clinical Practices in the Rising Costs of Hospital Care." *New England Journal of Medicine* 313 (1985):1201-08.

Thurow, Lester C. "Medicine Versus Economics." *New England Journal of Medicine* (1985):611-14.

Veatch, Robert M. "DRG's and the Ethical Allocation of Resources." *Hastings Center Report* 16 (June 1986):32-40.

Warner, Kenneth E., and Bryan R. Luce. *Cost-Benefit and Cost-Effectiveness Analysis in Health Care*. Ann Arbor, MI: Health Administration Press, 1982.

Wikler, Daniel. "Personal Responsibility for Illness." In *Health Care Ethics*, ed. Donald VanDeVeer and Tom Regan. Philadelphia: Temple University Press, 1987.

INDEX

admissions to health care settings, 52, 122-125, 130, 134-140. *See also* transfers from health care settings

advance directives, 6, 30, 39-40, 50, 63, 66, 69, 72, 75, 82, 83, 87-91, 96-97, 123

advance planning. *See* prospective planning *and* treatment plan

age as factor in decisionmaking, 38-41, 73

AIDS, 34-37

antibiotics, 65-69, 70-75, 92, 93

artificial feeding. *See* nutrition and hydration

autonomy. *See* self-determination

beneficence. *See* well-being

benefit
compared to cost, 31
compared to burden, 5, 12, 33, 36, 48, 61, 72, 73, 79, 82-83, 136, 140

best interests standard, 12, 35, 68, 73, 84, 89, 90, 103

bleeding, treatment for, 36, 46-50, 51-54. *See also* Jehovah's Witnesses *and* religious values and beliefs

blood transfusions. *See* bleeding, treatment for

brain death, 40, 101-104, 105-109, 121. *See also* death, declaration of *and* legislation

burden
compared to benefit, 5, 12, 30, 33, 48, 60, 61, 67, 71-72, 78, 82-83, 136, 140
to society. *See* social good

cancer, 3, 8-9, 11-12, 23, 43, 70, 76-77, 79, 81-84, 92-97, 122-125, 134-140

capacity, determinations of, 8-13, 19, 43, 45, 83, 90, 95, 96. *See also* decisionmaking

cardiac arrest. *See* resuscitation decisions

Cardiac Care Unit. *See* Intensive Care Unit

cardiopulmonary resuscitation (CPR). *See* DNR *and* resuscitation decisions *and* "Code" and "No Code"

challenges. *See* decisionmaking, review of *and* ethics committees

clergy, 11, 53, 55, 113-114, 118, 136

chronic obstructive lung disease, 3, 8, 17-18, 29, 32, 81-82, 126

"Code" and "No Code," 4, 38-41, 42, 93, 95, 113. *See also* DNR *and* resuscitation

comatose, 29, 34, 36, 59, 101, 113. *See also* irreversibly unconscious patients

comfort. *See* discomfort *and* pain relief *and* palliative care

communication
between patient and responsible health care professional, 3-7, 8-10, 23, 28, 30, 34-37, 39, 42-45, 46-50, 51-53, 76-80, 87-91, 92- 97, 126-129
between surrogate and responsible health care professional, 8-9, 11-12, 17-22, 55-58, 59-64, 65-69, 70-75, 87-91, 101-104, 113-117, 118-121, 122-125, 134-140
within health care team, 17-22, 51, 59-64, 93, 95, 114, 126-129, 134-140
See also surrogate, decisionmaking

competence. *See* capacity *and* decisionmaking

confidentiality, 114, 115

Coronary Care Unit. *See* Intensive Care Unit

cost containment, xiii, 31, 119, 130-133, 134-140. *See also* economic considerations

costs of care, xiii, 31, 122-125, 130-133, 134-140. *See also* economic considerations

costworthy care, 134-140. *See also* economic considerations

court review. *See* judicial review

death
declaration of, 101-104, 105-109
intended vs. foreseeable, 47-48, 74, 79, 82-83

decisionmaking
by patients with capacity, 11, 33, 36, 40, 72, 93, 96, 126-129, 136-137

157

Index

                                                                                          159

17-22, 23, 28, 31, 40, 42, 87, 93, 101, 103, 104, 113, 118, 126-129, 134-140
intubation, 9, 12, 18-19, 88, 91, 93, 127
irreversibly unconscious patients, 60, 61, 63, 89, 102, 118-121

Jehovah's Witnesses, 51-54. *See also* bleeding, treatment for *and* religious values and beliefs
judicial review, 25, 28, 52, 83, 84, 91, 96, 103, 117, 120
of decision about incapacity, 11, 13
of decision of surrogate, 13, 68, 90, 117, 120
of identification of surrogate, 83
justice, xiii, xv, 30-31, 33, 72, 91, 129, 130-133, 135, 136, 138. *See also* equity

killing, 19-20, 24- 25, 27, 56, 57, 60, 66, 74, 78, 84. 107. *See also* euthanasia *and* murder *and* death, intended vs. foreseeable

law, role of, 24- 28, 42, 45, 62, 67, 106, 108, 129. *See also* legislation
legal counsel, 9, 24-25, 27-28, 38, 104, 124
legislation, 102-103, 106-107, 108, 109, 122, 129. *See also* brain death *and* law, role of
"Living Will." *See* advance directive *and* treatment directive
long-term care facilities. *See* nursing homes

Medicaid, 124, 129, 130
Medicare, 124, 129
murder, 24, 27. *See also* euthanasia *and* killing

nasogastric tube, 55-56, 59, 60, 65, 72, 74, 113. *See also* nutrition and hydration
Nazis, xiii, 65, 66
No Code Orders. *See* "Code" *and* "No Code" *and* DNR
nurse, 21, 34, 38, 42, 45, 46, 47, 49, 59-64, 92, 102, 113-114, 116, 123, 126, 136
as responsible health care professional, 60, 123, 127-129
assisting in decisionmaking, 62, 113-114, 118
withdrawal from case, 50, 62. *See also* values, of health care professions

nursing homes, 8-13, 29, 32, 46-50, 55-58, 59-64, 70-75, 122, 126-129
as site of dying, 122, 125, 126-127
decisionmaking in, 8-13, 46-50, 55-58, 59-64, 70-75, 126-129
financial incentives of and reimbursement to, 122, 128-129
nutrition and hydration, 55-58, 59-64, 65, 72-74, 92. *See also* nasogastric tube

organ transplantation, 29, 31, 104, 106-107, 108, 109, 118, 120

pain medication, 20, 43, 79, 81-84, 92, 96
and acceleration of death, 79, 82-83
and addiction, 79, 83, 84
and unconsciousness, 84
pain relief, 43, 57, 65, 73, 79, 80, 81-84, 92
palliative care, xiii, 23, 28, 76-80, 81-84, 122, 123. *See also* discomfort *and* pain *and* suffering
patients' values and preferences. *See* decisionmaking *and* values, of patient
permanently unconscious patients. *See* irreversibly unconscious patients
persistent vegetative state (PVS). *See* irreversibly unconscious patients
physician, 3-7, 17-22, 23-24, 26-28, 34-37, 38, 42, 51, 55, 59, 61, 66, 76, 77, 83-84, 87-89, 94-95, 102-104, 105, 108, 113-117, 118, 122-123, 126-129, 130,132-133, 136-140
and ethics committee, 6, 9, 13, 50, 113-117, 118-121
as allocator of health care resources, 31-32, 132, 133, 135-137, 139
consultations and referrals, 51, 84, 114
decisionmaking for patients, 4, 88, 113-117, 126-127
relationship with patient, xiv, 24-26, 114-115, 133
withdrawal from case, 6, 50, 54, 69, 140.
See also values, of health care professions
pneumonia, 3, 8, 65- 69, 70- 75, 93
policy, xiii, 24, 28, 33, 41, 51-53, 60, 63, 72, 74, 83-84, 90, 93, 95-96, 103-104, 114, 116, 119, 121, 122-125, 126-129, 130-133, 134-140.
See also health care institutions
President's Commission for the Study of Ethical Problems in Medicine, 103